A BEGINNER'S GUIDE TO BLOOD CELLS

A Beginner's Guide to Blood Cells

2ⁿᵈ Edition

Barbara J. Bain

MB BS FRACP FRCPath
Reader in Diagnostic Haematology,
Department of Haematology
St Mary's Hospital Campus, Imperial College,
St Mary's Hospital,
London

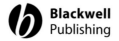
Blackwell
Publishing

© 1996, 2004 by Blackwell Publishing Ltd
Blackwell Publishing Inc., 350 Main Street, Malden, Massachusetts 02148-5020, USA
Blackwell Publishing Ltd, 9600 Garsington Road, Oxford OX4 2DQ, UK
Blackwell Science Asia Pty Ltd, 550 Swanston Street, Carlton, Victoria 3053, Australia

First published 1996
Second edition 2004
4   2007

Library of Congress Cataloging-in-Publication Data

Bain, Barbara J.
   A beginner's guide to blood cells / Barbara J. Bain.—2nd ed.
      p.   ;   cm.
   Includes index.
   ISBN 978-1-4051-2175-0
   1. Hematology–Handbooks, manuals, etc.   2. Blood cell–Handbooks, manuals, etc.
   [DNLM: 1. Blood Cells–physiology–Handbooks.   2. Blood Cells Count–methods–
Handbooks.   3. Blood Cells–pathology–Handbooks.   WH 39 B 162b 2004]   I. Title.

   RB45.B268   2004
   616.1'5–dc22

                                                              2004001756

ISBN: 978-1-4051-2175-0

A catalogue record for this title is available from the British Library

Set in 9.5 on 13 pt Trump by SNP Best-set Typesetter Ltd, Hong Kong
Printed and bound in India by Replika Press Pvt. Ltd

For further information on Blackwell Publishing, visit our website:
http:/www.blackwellpublishing.com

The publisher's policy is to use permanent paper from mills that operate a sustainable
forestry policy, and which has been manufactured from pulp processed using acid-
free and elementary chlorine-free practices. Furthermore, the publisher ensures that
the text paper and cover board used have met acceptable environmental accreditation
standards.

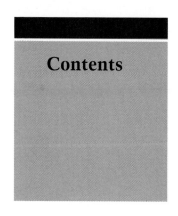

Contents

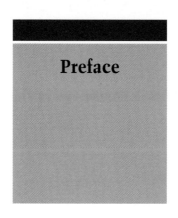

Preface

A Beginner's Guide to Blood Cells is an introduction to normal and abnormal blood cells and blood counts for trainees, whether they be trainee laboratory scientists, medical students, trainee haematologists or trainee physicians. It may be seen as complementary to *Blood Cells: a Practical Guide* (3rd Edn., Blackwell Science, Oxford, 2003), from which the illustrations are drawn. Unlike *Blood Cells*, *A Beginner's Guide* does not seek to be comprehensive. It introduces the important basic concepts, sets haematological findings in a clinical context and, in the final chapter, lets the reader test his or her own knowledge.

All photographs are of blood films stained by May–Grünwald–Giemsa (MGG) stain and all have been taken at the same magnification so that they can be readily compared with each other.

Barbara J. Bain
2004

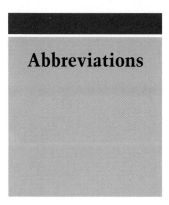

Abbreviations

dl	Decilitre
DNA	Deoxyribonucleic acid
FBC	Full blood count
fl	Femtolitre
G6PD	Glucose-6-phosphate dehydrogenase
Hb	Haemoglobin concentration
Hct	Haematocrit
HDW	Haemoglobin distribution width
MCH	Mean cell haemoglobin
MCHC	Mean cell haemoglobin concentration
MCV	Mean cell volume
MGG	May–Grünwald–Giemsa
HPLC	High performance liquid chromatography
NRBC	Nucleated red blood cell
PCV	Packed cell volume
pg	Picogram
RBC	Red blood cell count
RDW	Red cell distribution width
RNA	Ribonucleic acid
WBC	White blood cell count

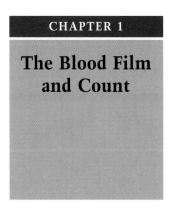

The Blood Film and Count

Blood

Blood is a life-sustaining fluid which circulates through the heart and blood vessels. It carries oxygen and nutrients to the tissues and waste products to the lungs, liver and kidneys, where they can be removed from the body. Usually when blood is removed from the body it forms a solid blood clot. However, if clotting is prevented by mixing with an anticoagulant, the blood separates, under the influence of gravity, into three layers (Fig. 1.1). The bottom layer is deep red in colour and is composed of red cells. The top layer is clear and pale yellow. It is called plasma and is composed of various salts and proteins dissolved in water. In between is a narrow layer called the buffy coat because of its buff or yellowish white colour. The buffy coat is composed mainly of cells of a variety of types, collectively known as white cells. In addition there are small cellular fragments, called platelets, which have a role in blood clotting.

The blood film

Although we can judge the proportions of red cells and white cells in a tube of sedimented blood, we get far more information if the blood is carefully mixed and a thin layer is spread on a glass slide to form a blood film. The blood cells are then preserved by exposure to the alcohol methanol, a process known as fixation. The fixed film of blood is stained with a mixture of several dyes so that the individual cells can be recognized when they are examined with a microscope. After staining, the colour of red

1

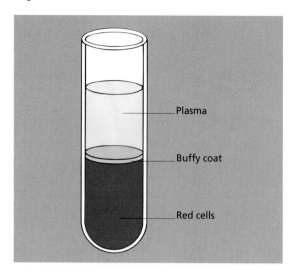

Fig. 1.1 Diagram of a tube of anticoagulated blood which has been allowed to sediment, showing the separation of blood into red cells, a buffy coat (white cells and platelets) and plasma.

cells is enhanced and the white cells and platelets, which would otherwise be transparent and colourless, have acquired a variety of colours which allow their detailed structure to be recognized. One of the commonest mixtures of dyes used to stain blood cells is the May–Grünwald–Giemsa (MGG) stain, named after its inventors. All the photographs in this book are of MGG-stained blood films.

Red cells

The most numerous cells in a blood film are the red cells, also known as erythrocytes. Normal red cells are disc-shaped but are thinner in the centre (Fig. 1.2). As a consequence, on a stained blood film, they have a circular outline and a paler central area (Fig. 1.3). Red cells owe their pinkish-brown colour to the presence of a complex protein, haemoglobin, which is their major constituent. Enhancement of their colour in a stained film is because haemoglobin takes up eosin, one of the dyes of the MGG stain. In the body it is haemoglobin of the red cells which, in the

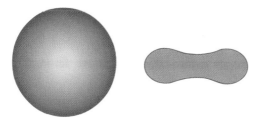

Fig. 1.2 A diagram of a red cell viewed from above and in cross-section.

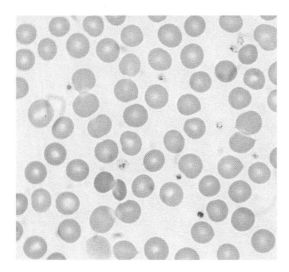

Fig. 1.3 Normal red cells (erythrocytes) showing little variation in size and shape, an approximately round outline and a small area of central pallor in some of the cells. The small lilac-staining structures between the red cells are platelets.

lungs, combines with oxygen from inspired air and transports it to tissues where it is needed for the metabolic processes supplying the energy needs of the body. Mature red cells in humans (although not in some other species) differ from most body cells in that they do not have a nucleus. Red cells are produced in the bone marrow and usually lose their nuclei when they are released into the blood stream.

White cells

In healthy people there are at least five types of white cell or leucocyte in the circulating blood. Unlike red cells, white cells have retained their nuclei. The cell is therefore made up of a nucleus and cytoplasm. The cytoplasm is the site of protein synthesis and other cellular functions. The nucleus is composed of chromatin, which is mainly deoxyribonucleic

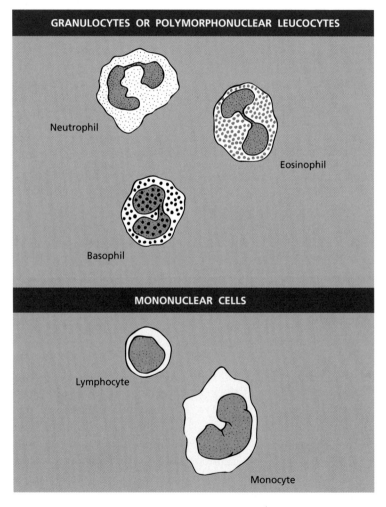

Fig. 1.4 A diagram showing how white cells are classified.

acid (DNA), carrying genetic messages. Genetic messages are transmitted from the nucleus to the cytoplasm by ribonucleic acid (RNA).

White cells are divided into granulocytes (also known as polymorphonuclear leucocytes) and mononuclear cells. There are three types of granulocyte and two types of mononuclear cell (Fig. 1.4). The names are not very logical but they have been in use for a long time and are generally accepted. Granulocytes are so named because their cytoplasm contains prominent granules. However, monocytes also have granules and so do some lymphocytes. The term polymorphonuclear leucocyte refers to the very variable nuclear shape which is typical of granulocytes. The term mononuclear cell means that the cell has only a single nucleus. However, this is true of granulocytes, as well as of the cells conventionally referred to as mononuclear. The functions of the various leucocytes are summarized in Table 1.1.

Neutrophils

Neutrophils (Fig. 1.5) have a nucleus which stains purple and is divided into two to five segments or lobes. The lobes are separated by a thin strand or filament of nuclear material. The nuclear chromatin is heterogeneous with some clumping. The cytoplasm of neutrophils is very pale blue and is packed with fine lilac-staining granules. The granules are referred to as

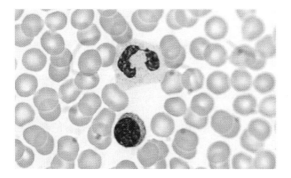

Fig. 1.5 A normal neutrophil with a bilobed nucleus and cytoplasm containing delicate lilac-staining granules. The other nucleated cell is a small lymphocyte.

Table 1.1 The functions of leucocytes.

Cell	Major function		
Neutrophil	Is attracted to sites of infection by a process known as chemotaxis; ingests micro-organisms (a process known as phagocytosis) and destroys them		
Eosinophil	The same functions as the neutrophil; in addition, helps control parasitic infections; has a role in allergic responses		
Basophil	Has a role in immediate hypersensitivity reactions, allergic and inflammatory responses and in the control of parasitic infections		
Lymphocyte	Mediates immune responses	B lymphocyte matures into a plasma cell, which secretes antibodies (humoral immunity)	
		T lymphocyte attacks cells bearing foreign antigens and antibody-coated cells; can help or suppress B cells (part of cell-mediated immunity)	
		Natural killer lymphocyte (NK cell) attacks foreign cells and tumour cells (part of cell-mediated immunity)	
Monocyte	Phagocytoses and kills micro-organisms including mycobacteria and fungi, phagocytoses cells or organisms that have bound immunoglobulin or complement and phagocytoses dead and damaged cells; presents antigen to cells of the immune system; migrates to tissues where it differentiates, to become a long-lived phagocytic and antigen-presenting cell known as a macrophage		

neutrophilic because they owe their colour to uptake of both the acidic and the basic components of the stain. In females a proportion of the neutrophils have a very small lobe, known as a 'drumstick', protruding from the nucleus (Fig. 1.6). It represents the inactive X-chromosome of the cell.

Neutrophils are produced in the bone marrow. They spend 6–10 hours in the blood stream before moving from capillaries into tissues. The major function of neutrophils is as tissue phagocytes. They move preferentially to sites of infection or inflammation where they ingest, kill and break down bacteria. The process of moving to sites of infection or inflammation

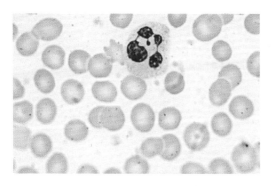

Fig. 1.6 A normal neutrophil from a female showing a nucleus with four lobes and a 'drumstick'.

is known as chemotaxis and occurs in response to activated complement components and chemical signals released by a variety of cells. The process of ingesting bacteria is known as phagocytosis.

Eosinophils

Eosinophils (Fig. 1.7) have a nucleus that is usually bilobed and pale blue cytoplasm, which is packed with large refractile, orange–red granules. The granules are referred to as eosinophilic because they take up the acidic dye eosin. Eosinophils are produced in the bone marrow and circulate in the blood stream for

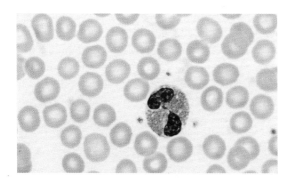

Fig. 1.7 A normal bilobed eosinophil. The granules are reddish-orange and pack the cytoplasm.

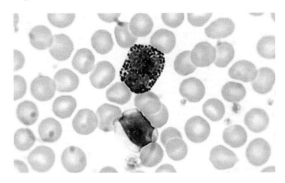

Fig. 1.8 A normal basophil. The nucleus has three lobes. The cytoplasm is packed with large purple granules. (The lower cell is a lymphocyte.)

about 6 hours before migrating to tissues. They respond to chemotactic stimuli, are phagocytic and can kill ingested organisms. They are important in the body's defences against tissue parasites, being able to discharge their granule contents extracellularly, seriously damaging large parasites. Eosinophils are also involved in allergic reactions.

Basophils

Basophils (Fig. 1.8) have a lobulated nucleus, which is often obscured by the large purple-staining granules which pack the very pale blue cytoplasm. The granules are referred to as basophilic because they take up basic components of the stain (such as methylene blue). In fact they stain metachromatically with basic stains, i.e. the granules react with a blue dye to produce a purple colour. Basophils are produced in the bone marrow and circulate in the blood in small numbers before migrating to tissue. They have a role in allergic and inflammatory responses.

Lymphocytes

Lymphocytes are the second most numerous circulating white cell after neutrophils. They are smaller than granulocytes with a round or somewhat irregular outline and pale blue, clear

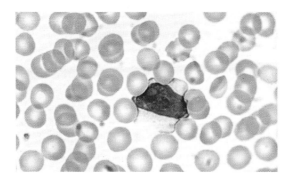

Fig. 1.9 A large lymphocyte with a less densely staining nucleus than occurs in a small lymphocyte and more plentiful pale blue cytoplasm. A nucleolus is apparent, top left in the nucleus.

cytoplasm. Some lymphocytes have a variable number of azurophilic (pinkish-purple) granules. Lymphocytes are divided into three morphological categories, depending on their size, the amount of cytoplasm and the presence or absence of cytoplasmic granules. These categories are small lymphocyte (Fig. 1.5), large lymphocyte (Fig. 1.9) and large granular lymphocyte (Fig. 1.10). Small lymphocytes are most numerous. The nuclear chromatin of lymphocytes may be dense and homogeneous (particularly in small lymphocytes) or more lightly staining and somewhat heterogeneous (particularly in large lymphocytes).

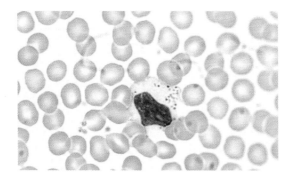

Fig. 1.10 A large granular lymphocyte showing a moderate number of prominent azurophilic granules in clear cytoplasm.

Occasional normal lymphocytes show a discrete but ill-defined paler structure within the nucleus, which is the nucleolus.

Lymphocytes are produced from lymphoid stem cells in the bone marrow and probably the thymus. Their function is in tissues such as lymph nodes, spleen, tonsils and the lymphoid tissue associated with mucous membranes. They circulate in the blood stream, enter lymphoid tissues and emerge again from lymphoid tissues into lymphatic channels, where they form one constituent of a clear fluid known as lymph. Lymphatics drain into the thoracic duct and ultimately into the blood stream. This process of continuing movement between tissues and the blood stream is known as lymphocyte recirculation. Lymphocytes function in the body's immune responses. They are divided into three functional types: B cells, T cells and natural killer (NK) cells. B cells differentiate in tissues into plasma cells, which secrete antibodies, thereby providing humoral immunity. T cells function in cell-mediated immunity as do NK cells. T cells also modulate B cell function. The functional categories of lymphocyte show little correlation with morphological categories except that large granular lymphocytes are either T cells or NK cells. However, other T cells cannot be distinguished morphologically from B cells. The functional categories of lymphocytes are of far more importance than the morphological categories.

Monocytes

Monocytes (Fig. 1.11) are the largest normal blood cells. They have lobulated nuclei and voluminous cytoplasm which is greyish-blue, is sometimes opaque and may be vacuolated or contain fine azurophilic granules.

Monocytes have an intravascular life span of several days. They function mainly in tissues where they differentiate into long-lived macrophages (sometimes called histiocytes). Monocytes and macrophages respond to chemotactic stimuli and are phagocytic. They are part of the body's defences against bacterial and fungal infections and also ingest and break down dead and dying body cells. They present antigen to lymphocytes.

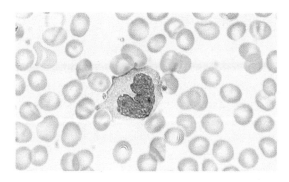

Fig. 1.11 A monocyte, showing a lobulated nucleus and voluminous, opaque cytoplasm containing very fine azurophilic granules. Several platelets are also visible. (Monocytes should not be confused with large granular lymphocytes. Lymphocytes have clear, pale blue cytoplasm and discrete, sometimes prominent granules whereas monocytes usually have more opaque, grey–blue cytoplasm with very fine granules.)

They secrete chemical messengers, known as cytokines, which influence the behaviour of other body cells, including blood cells and their precursors. Monocytes differentiate not only into macrophages but also into various specialized cells, specific to different organs, such as the Kupffer cells of the liver and the microglial cells of the brain.

Platelets

Platelets are produced within the vascular channels (sinusoids) of the bone marrow by the fragmentation of the protruding cytoplasm of large bone marrow cells known as megakaryocytes. They are thus not, strictly speaking, cells but rather are fragments of the cytoplasm of cells.

Platelets are considerably smaller than red cells and white cells (Fig. 1.11). They are pale blue with fine azurophilic granules which tend to be clustered in the centre of the platelet. When blood films are made, as is generally the case, from anticoagulated blood, the platelets are usually discrete and separate from each other, but in some circumstances they form clumps or aggregates.

Haemopoietic cells

Peripheral blood cells are produced in the bone marrow. Their precursors are referred to as haemopoietic cells (Fig. 1.12). The only significant function of haemopoietic cells is the production of mature end cells. Recognizable haemopoietic precursors are present in the circulating blood of healthy subjects but, except in the neonatal period and during pregnancy, they are quite uncommon and are not often noted in a blood film. They are much commoner in patients with leukaemia or other haematological disorders and in patients with severe infection or other serious systemic diseases.

Myeloblasts

Myeloblasts (Fig. 1.13) are very rare in the blood of healthy subjects. They are larger than lymphocytes but often smaller than monocytes. They have a high nucleocytoplasmic ratio and scanty to moderate amounts of cytoplasm, which varies from weakly to moderately basophilic. (Basophilic in this context indicates a blue colour consequent on the uptake of basic dyes.) The nucleus is approximately round, nuclear chromatin is diffuse and nucleoli may be apparent. In patients with leukaemia and related disorders, the cytoplasm may contain small numbers of azurophilic granules or other inclusions or vacuoles (see page 91). Myeloblasts are precursors of neutrophils, eosinophils and basophils.

Promyelocytes

Promyelocytes (Fig. 1.14) are rare in the blood of healthy people. They are larger than myeloblasts with more plentiful cytoplasm and consequently a lower nucleocytoplasmic ratio. The cytoplasm is more basophilic than that of a myeloblast and contains azurophilic (pinkish-purple) primary granules. Sometimes there is a more lightly staining zone in the cytoplasm adjacent to the nucleus, which represents the Golgi apparatus, where granules are produced. The nucleus is round or oval, is usually eccentric, shows some chromatin condensation and has a

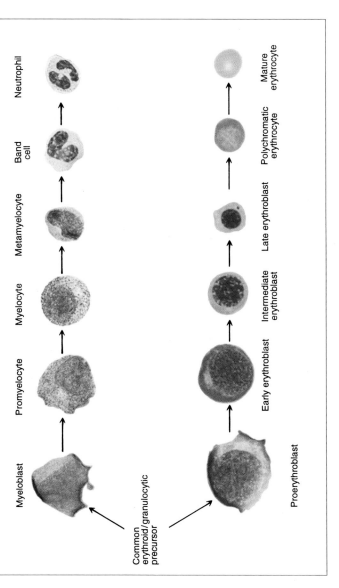

Fig. 1.12 A diagram showing the relationship of haemopoietic precursors to each other and to the end cells into which they differentiate. Proliferation of cells occurs simultaneously with maturation or differentiation so that one myeloblast is likely to give rise to 16 mature granulocytes and one proerythroblast to 16 red cells. Myeloblasts, promyelocytes and myelocytes are all cells capable of cell division or mitosis. Metamyelocytes and all later cells are non-dividing cells. All red cell precursors with the exception of late erythroblasts are dividing cells. Myeloblasts differentiate not only into neutrophils, as shown in the diagram, but also into eosinophils and basophils.

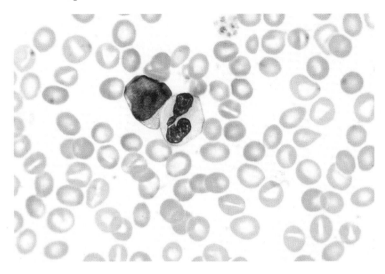

Fig. 1.13 A blood film of a patient showing a myeloblast and a neutrophil. The myeloblast has a high nucleocytoplasmic ratio, a diffuse chromatin pattern and a single nucleolus. The neutrophil is hypogranular.

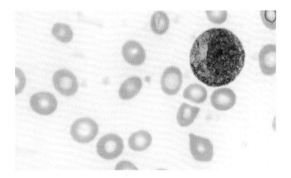

Fig. 1.14 A promyelocyte showing a lower nucleocytoplasmic ratio than that of a myeloblast, an eccentric nucleus, azurophilic granules and a Golgi zone to the left of the nucleus.

visible nucleolus. Because they have no specific (lineage-associated) granules, promyelocytes, which are precursors of neutrophils, eosinophils or basophils, cannot generally be distinguished from each other.

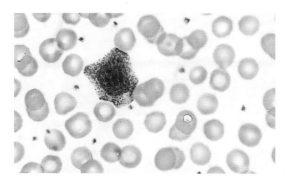

Fig. 1.15 A neutrophil myelocyte showing a smaller cell than a promyelocyte with some condensation of nuclear chromatin and no visible nucleolus. On microscopic examination it is apparent that such cells have primary and secondary granules with different staining characteristics.

Myelocytes

Myelocytes (Fig. 1.15) are uncommon in the blood of healthy subjects except in the neonatal period and during pregnancy. They are smaller than promyelocytes. They have not only azurophilic or primary granules but also secondary granules characteristic of specific lineages, i.e. neutrophilic, eosinophilic or basophilic granules. The myelocyte nucleus is round or oval and shows chromatin condensation; no nucleolus is apparent.

Metamyelocytes

Small numbers of neutrophil metamyelocytes (Fig. 1.16) are present in the blood of healthy subjects. Basophil and eosinophil metamyelocytes are not seen in the blood of healthy subjects. Metamyelocytes have similar characteristics to myelocytes but differ in that the nucleus is indented, U-shaped or C-shaped and the primary granules are usually no longer apparent.

Band cells

Neutrophil band forms (Fig. 1.17) are present as a minor population in the blood of healthy people. They are intermediate in characteristics between metamyelocytes and mature

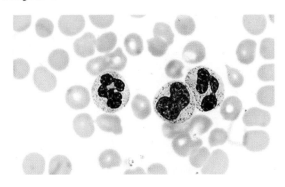

Fig. 1.16 A neutrophil metamyelocyte between two segmented neutrophils. The nucleus is indented.

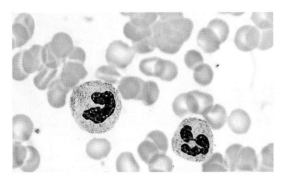

Fig. 1.17 A neutrophil band form (left) compared with a segmented neutrophil (right).

neutrophils. The nucleus has an irregular shape with some parallel edges so that it resembles a band or ribbon. It differs from a mature or segmented neutrophil in that the nucleus is not divided into distinct lobes or segments. Eosinophil and basophil band forms are quite uncommon.

Nucleated red blood cells

Nucleated red blood cells (NRBC) or erythroblasts (Fig. 1.18) are present in very small numbers in healthy people, except during the neonatal period. Those which are most likely to be released

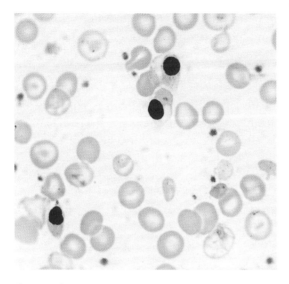

Fig. 1.18 Three nucleated red blood cells (NRBC) showing a small densely staining nucleus and cytoplasm which is pink because of the presence of haemoglobin.

into the blood stream are late erythroblasts. They can be readily recognized because the cytoplasm is at least partly haemoglobinized giving them a pinkish or lilac tinge. NRBC have a superficial resemblance to lymphocytes but can be distinguished from them not only by the colour of the cytoplasm but also by the lower nucleocytoplasmic ratio and the denser, more homogeneously staining nucleus.

The blood count

Haematology laboratories not only examine blood films. They also perform various measurements relating to the haemoglobin content of the blood, the characteristics of red cells and the number of red cells, white cells and platelets. These measurements are collectively referred to as a blood count or full blood count (FBC). During illness, abnormalities can develop in any of the cells in the blood. The purpose of performing a blood count and examining a blood film is to detect quantitative and qualitative abnormalities in blood cells. Their detection often helps in diagnosis and in the treatment of the patient.

Haemoglobin concentration

If red cells are lysed, the haemoglobin is released from the red cells and forms a solution in the plasma. The haemoglobin concentration (Hb) can be measured biochemically by light absorption at a specified wave length after a chemical reaction which converts haemoglobin to cyanmethaemoglobin or to lauryl sulphate haemoglobin. Hb is measured in either grams per decilitre (g/dl) or grams per litre (g/l). A fall in the Hb is referred to as anaemia.

Haematocrit or packed cell volume

An alternative way of detecting anaemia is to centrifuge a tube containing an aliquot of blood and measure the proportion of the column of blood which is occupied by the red cells. Nowadays an equivalent measurement is made by various automated instruments using a quite different principle to get the same information. This test is called a packed cell volume (PCV) or a haematocrit (Hct). Some haematologists use these two terms interchangeably while others used PCV to refer to a measurement made after centrifugation and Hct for an estimate made by an automated instrument. This measurement is expressed as a decimal percentage, i.e. as litres/litre (e.g. 0.45).

Cell counts

Traditionally blood cells were counted by diluting a small quantity of blood in a diluent which could also stain the cells or, if white cells or platelets were to be counted, could lyse the more numerous red cells. The diluted blood was placed in a counting chamber of known volume and the number of cells present was counted microscopically. Such a method of counting blood cells is very labour-intensive and not suited to the large number of blood counts needed in modern medical practice. Nowadays blood cells are counted by large automated instruments.

A stream of cells in a diluent passes through a sensing zone. They are sensed either because they pass through an electric field or because they pass through a beam of light. Each cell passing through the sensing zone generates an electrical impulse, which can then be counted. Red cells are both relatively large and relatively numerous and so can be readily counted. White cells can be counted by lysing the more numerous red cells or by altering the red cells in some way so that they are 'invisible' to the instrument. Platelets are distinguished from other cells by their smaller size. Cell counts are expressed as the number of cells in a litre of blood. The red blood cell count (RBC) is expressed as a number $\times 10^{12}$ per litre (e.g. 5×10^{12}/l). The white blood cell count (WBC) and platelet count are expressed as a number $\times 10^9$ per litre (e.g. 7.5×10^9/l and 140×10^9/l). A white cell count of 7.5×10^9/l means that there are 7 500 000 000 cells in a litre of blood.

Red cell indices

Red cells can vary in their size and in the amount of haemoglobin contained in an individual cell. Abnormalities in both these cell characteristics are common in certain inherited abnormalities and when people are sick. Diagnostically useful information can be obtained by measuring them. Traditionally the size of red cells was estimated by dividing the PCV by the number of cells in the blood to give a mean cell volume (MCV). The haemoglobin content of individual cells was estimated by dividing the Hb by the RBC to give a mean cell haemoglobin (MCH). The Hb of individual cells was estimated by dividing the Hb by the PCV to give a mean cell haemoglobin concentration (MCHC). Nowadays, not only is the PCV estimated electronically but the size of a red cell can be calculated from the height of the electrical impulse which is generated when the cell passes through a light beam or through an electrical field. As the automated instruments also measure the total Hb of the blood, it is a simple matter for the red cell indices to be produced automatically as part of the blood count. Instruments can be designed to measure the MCV and calculate the PCV/Hct from the MCV and the RBC or, alternatively, to measure the PCV/Hct and calculate the MCV from the PCV/Hct and the RBC. The formulae which relate the various red cell indices to each other are as follows:

$$MCV = \frac{PCV\left(l/l\right) \times 1000}{RBC\left(cells/l\right) \times 10^{-12}} \qquad (1)$$

e.g. if the PCV is 0.33 and the RBC 4.1 × 10¹²/l, then

$$MCV = \frac{0.33 \times 1000}{4.1} = 80.5\,fl\left(femtolitres\right)$$

(In understanding this formula and the following ones, it should be noted that if the RBC is 4.1 × 10¹²/l then 4.1 is the RBC/l × 10⁻¹².)

$$MCH = \frac{Hb\left(g/dl\right) \times 10}{RBC\left(cells/l\right) \times 10^{-12}} \qquad (2)$$

e.g. if the Hb is 12.3 g/dl and the RBC is 4.1 × 10¹²/l then

$$MCH = \frac{12.3 \times 10}{4.1} = 30\ pg\left(picograms\right)$$

$$MCHC = \frac{Hb\left(g/dl\right)}{PCV\left(l/l\right)} \qquad (3)$$

e.g. if the Hb is 12.3 g/dl and the PCV/Hct is 0.33 then

$$MCHC = \frac{12.3}{0.33} = 37.3\,g/dl$$

If an instrument measures the RBC rather than the PCV/Hct, then the formula is

$$RBC/l \times 10^{-12} = \frac{PCV\left(l/l\right) \times 1000}{MCV\left(fl\right)} \qquad (4)$$

e.g. using the same figures as above

$$RBC/l \times 10^{-12} = \frac{0.33 \times 1000}{80.5} = 4.1$$

Normal ranges

In order to interpret blood counts it is necessary to know what is normal. This is usually done by reference to either a normal range or a reference range. A reference range is more strictly defined than a normal range but both represent the range of test results which would be expected in healthy people of the same age and sex (and, if relevant, of the same ethnic origin) as the person being investigated. Conventionally, both types of range are expressed as the central 95% of test results that would be expected in healthy people. The reason for excluding the top 2.5% and the bottom 2.5% is that there is usually an overlap between test results of healthy people and of those who are sick. A 95% range has been chosen to avoid either classifying too many healthy subjects as abnormal or missing relevant abnormalities in patients who are sick. It is clear that for any one test 5% of healthy subjects will have results falling outside the 'normal' range. Conversely, a patient who is sick may have a test result which is abnormal for him or her but which is still within the normal range. For example, a man may have a large gastrointestinal haemorrhage, causing his Hb to fall from its normal level of around 16 g/dl to 14 g/dl. The latter – 14 g/dl – is within the range expected for a healthy adult man but for this particular patient it is abnormal. This is because the range of test results expected in a group of healthy people is much wider than the range expected if the same test is repeated day after day in the same person. Usually we have no way of knowing what is 'normal' for a particular individual and so we have to resort to comparing his or her test results with a normal range.

The statistical distribution of test results differs for different tests. Many tests, e.g. the Hb, show a normal or Gaussian distribution. This means that if the distribution of the test results is plotted on graph paper a bell-shaped curve is obtained (Fig. 1.19a). If this is so, the 95% range can be calculated by estimating the mean ± 2 standard deviations. Other test results, e.g. the WBC (Fig. 1.19b), have a skewed distribution which only becomes bell-shaped if the test results are plotted on logarithmic graph paper. Test results with this type of distribution require special statistical treatment to derive the normal range.

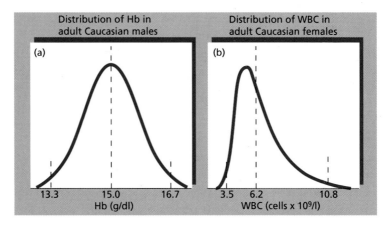

Fig. 1.19 Smoothed histograms showing (a) the normal distribution of Hb and (b) the log normal distribution of the white cell count.

Some normal ranges applicable to healthy people are shown in Tables 1.2–1.4. However, it should be noted that the test results for some haematological variables, e.g. the MCV, vary according to the method of measurement and it is desirable for laboratories to derive their own normal ranges for their own automated instruments by obtaining blood samples from a large number of healthy people. In the case of children, it is always difficult to obtain blood samples from large numbers of healthy individuals of various ages. As a consequence, published normal ranges for children are not as reliable as those for adults.

How to examine a blood film

Blood films should be examined in a systematic way. First the film should be examined without using the microscope, to make sure it is well spread (not too thick, too long or too short) and that its staining characteristics are normal. A film that is a deeper blue than other films stained in the same batch is usually indicative of an increase in the concentration of plasma proteins. This can be diagnostically important since it is often caused by multiple myeloma (a plasma cell malignancy) (see page 87) or by chronic inflammatory disease.

Table 1.2 Normal ranges for healthy Caucasian adults.

	Males	**Females**
WBC × 10⁻⁹/l	3.7–9.5	3.9–11.1
RBC × 10⁻¹²/l	4.32–5.66	3.88–4.99
Hb (g/dl)	13.3–16.7	11.8–14.8
PCV (Hct) (l/l)	0.39–0.5	0.36–0.44
MCV (fl)	82–98	
MCH (pg)	27.3–32.6	
MCHC (g/dl)	31.6–34.9	
RDW	9.5–15.5*	
	11.6–13.9†	
HDW	1.82–2.64†	
Neutrophils × 10⁻⁹/l	1.7–6.1	1.7–7.5
Lymphocytes × 10⁻⁹/l	1.0–3.2	
Monocytes × 10⁻⁹/l	0.2–0.6	
Eosinophils × 10⁻⁹/l	0.03–0.06	
Basophils × 10⁻⁹/l	0.02–0.29	
Large unstained cells (LUC) × 10⁻⁹/l	0.09–0.29	
Platelets × 10⁻⁹/l	143–332	169–358

RDW, red cell distribution width; HDW, haemoglobin distribution width.
The differential white cell counts and the platelet counts are for
Technicon H.1 series automated instruments. The ranges are wider for
manual differential counts, particularly for monocytes, eosinophils and
basophils. Platelet counts are very dependent on the method used for
counting and should be assessed only in relation to a normal range derived
for the instrument or method in use.
* Coulter S Plus IV.
† Technicon H.1 series.

Next the film is examined microscopically at low power (e.g.
with a ×25 objective) so that a large part of the film can be
scanned rapidly to detect any abnormal cells present in small
numbers. Finally the film is examined at a higher power (e.g.
with a ×40 or ×50 objective) so that the detailed structure of cells
can be assessed. The great majority of films can be evaluated
perfectly adequately without using high power (i.e. a ×100 oil
immersion objective). High power can be reserved for making a
detailed assessment of films that show significant abnormalities
requiring further assessment. In examining a film be sure to look

Table 1.3 Normal ranges for Afro-Caribbean and Africans for those haematological variables where the ranges differ from those of Caucasians.

	Males	Females
West Indians		
WBC × 10^{-9}/l	2.8–9.5	3.3–9.8
Neutrophils × 10^{-9}/l	1.0–5.8	1.4–6.5
Platelets × 10^{-9}/l	122–313	149–374
Africans		
WBC × 10^{-9}/l	2.8–7.2	3.2–7.8
Neutrophils × 10^{-9}/l	0.9–4.2	1.3–4.2
Platelets × 10^{-9}/l	115–290	125–342

It should be noted that the lower RBC, Hb, PCV and MCV observed in Afro-Caribbean and Africans are likely to be consequent on a high prevalence of thalassaemia trait and haemoglobinopathies rather than on other ethnic differences. It is therefore appropriate to use Caucasian reference ranges for red cell variables for Afro-Caribbean and Africans.

Table 1.4 Approximate 95% ranges for red cell variables and for automated* total and differential white cell counts for Caucasian infants and children.

Age (years)	RBC (× 10^{12}/l)	Hb (g/dl)	MCV (fl)
Birth	3.5–6.7	14–24	100–135
1	4.1–5.3	11–14	71–84
2–5	4.2–5.0	11–14	73–86
6–9	4.3–5.1	11–14	75–88
9–12	4.3–5.1	11.5–15.5	76–91

Age (years)	WBC	Neutrophil count	Lymphocyte count	Monocyte count	Eosinophil count
Birth	5–23	1.7–19	1–11	0.1–3.5	0.05–2
1	5.6–17.5	1.5–7	2.5–9	0.15–1.3	0.06–0.6
2–5	5–13	1.5–8.5	1.5–5.5†	0.15–1.3	0.08–1.2
6–9	4–10	1.5–6	1.5–4	0.15–1.3	0.08–1
9–12	4–10	1.5–6	1.5–4	0.15–1.3	0.04–0.8

* Ranges will be wider for manual differential counts than for automated counts.
† The lymphocyte count is up to 8 × 10^9/l in 2-year-olds, up to 5.5 × 10^9/l in 3- and 4-year-olds and up to 4.5 × 10^9/l in 5-year-olds.

specifically at red cells, white cells and platelets so that no abnormality is inadvertently overlooked. Be sure to look at the edges and tail of the film where abnormal cells may be found.

Finally, decide if a differential count is needed. Nowadays this will often have been performed by an automated instrument but you may need to verify its accuracy and in leukaemia you may need to carry out a manual differential count, i.e. one performed with the aid of a microscope.

Learning to look at blood films

When learning to recognize cells for the first time it is useful to compare cells seen down the microscope with photographs. Examining films on a double-headed microscope with an experienced laboratory worker is also very valuable. To learn to recognize high and low WBC and platelet counts, start by comparing the film appearance with the count on an automated instrument. After you have had some experience try to estimate what the count will be before you look at the test results. Later you will need to be able to do this fairly accurately so that you can recognize erroneous instrument counts. Similarly, start by looking at films with high and low MCVs and compare the size of the red cells with neutrophils and lymphocytes until you can recognize large and small red cells. When you have had some experience try to estimate the approximate MCV before you look at the test results. Eventually you will be able to judge the MCV, at least to within 5–10 fl.

Recognizing problems with the blood sample

Before carrying out a detailed assessment of a blood film it is important to detect any abnormal characteristics of the specimen which might interfere with your assessment of the film or with the accuracy of the automated count. The most common problem is storage artefact (Fig. 1.20). This occurs when blood has been at room temperature for a day or more before reaching the laboratory. The red cells turn into echinocytes, i.e. their shape alters so that the surface is covered with numerous short, regular projections. This process is also known as crenation.

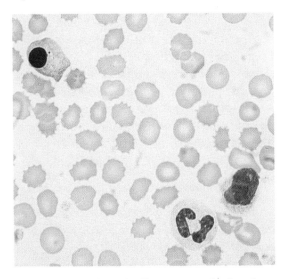

Fig. 1.20 Storage artefact. The red cells are crenated, a lymphocyte (right) has a fuzzy outline and one of the two neutrophils (left) has a nucleus which has become round, dense and homogeneous. (Compare the degenerating neutrophil with the nucleated red cells shown in Fig. 1.18.)

Some of the white cells develop fuzzy outlines or disintegrate entirely when the blood film is spread. The nuclei of neutrophils become dense, homogeneous and round and may break up into two or more round masses. It is important not to confuse these degenerating neutrophils with NRBC. They have a lower nucleo-cytoplasmic ratio and the cytoplasm is pink and slightly granular rather than reddish-brown. It is impossible to give any reliable opinion of films showing storage artefact. If the blood count is normal they can usually be ignored but if there is any reason to suspect a haematological abnormality a fresh blood sample must be obtained.

A common cause of inaccurate blood counts is partial clotting of the specimen or aggregation of the platelets. Platelets may aggregate because they have been activated (i.e. the process of blood clotting has started) or because there is an antibody present in the plasma which leads to platelet aggregation in blood that is anticoagulated with ethylenediaminetetra-acetic acid (EDTA). Aggregated platelets form masses between the red cells, that may contain intact platelets (Fig. 1.21) or may be composed of totally degranulated platelets, which stain pale blue. Less often, partially clotted samples contain fibrin strands, which are seen as pale blue or almost non-staining linear structures running between and deforming red cells (Fig. 1.22). Another *in vitro* artefact, less common than platelet aggregation but which can also lead to falsely low platelet counts, is platelet satellitism (Fig. 1.23).

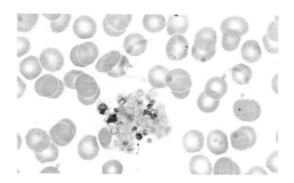

Fig. 1.21 A platelet aggregate containing a mixture of intact and degranulated platelets.

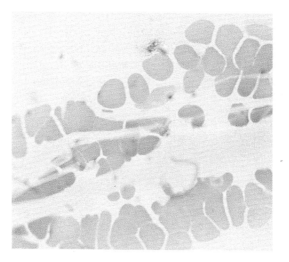

Fig. 1.22 Fibrin strands passing between and over red cells.

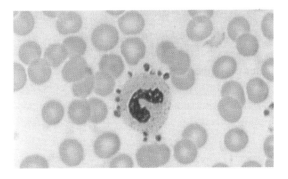

Fig. 1.23 Platelet satellitism.

Less common artefacts which should be recognized are those due to accidental freezing or overheating of the blood specimen before it reaches the laboratory and the presence of lipid (fat) in the plasma. All these abnormalities cause anomalous blood counts.

Interpreting blood films

When assessing blood films, always note the age, sex and ethnic origin of the patient and keep in mind what would be normal for that individual. Also consider the clinical details so that you can look carefully for any specific abnormalities which might be relevant, keeping in mind that the clinical details may provide you with an obvious explanation for an abnormality you have noted. For example, if the clinical details were 'alcohol excess' you would not be surprised to find that the patient had macrocytosis and you would go on to see if there were stomatocytes or any of the other abnormalities which could be caused by alcohol. Your report of these abnormalities would give the clinician very specific information which would help to confirm his/her clinical suspicion.

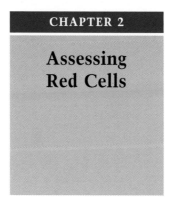

CHAPTER 2

Assessing Red Cells

Red cells should be assessed as to their:
- number
- size
- shape
- degree of haemoglobinization
- distribution in the blood film.

Their appearance should be described using a standard terminology.

Assessing red cell number and distribution (anaemia, polycythaemia, rouleaux formation, red cell agglutination)

The thickness of a film of blood spread on a glass slide is determined by how thick the blood is, i.e. by its viscosity. This in turn is determined by the Hb. In a normal blood film it is possible to find a part of the film which is ideal for microscopic examination where the red cells are touching but not overlapping. If the Hb is abnormally high (a condition referred to as polycythaemia) the blood has a high viscosity and the film of blood on the glass slide is thick. The red cells therefore appear packed together throughout the whole length of the film. The term 'packed film' is often used. Conversely, when a patient is anaemic the viscosity of the blood is low, the blood film is very thin and there are large spaces between the red cells. The effect of Hb on the blood film can be seen by comparing Figs 2.1, 2.2 and 2.3.

Usually red cells are distributed fairly regularly on the slide. Two abnormalities of distribution may occur. When there is an

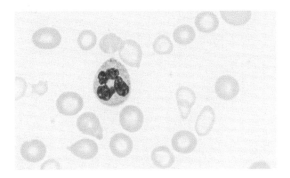

Fig. 2.1 Anaemia (caused by iron deficiency).

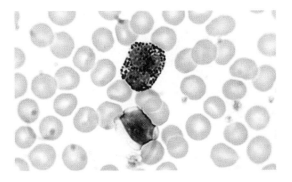

Fig. 2.2 Normal distribution of red cells in a healthy subject with normal Hb.

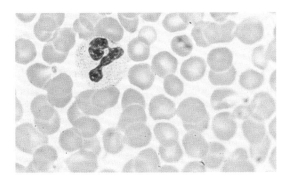

Fig. 2.3 Polycythaemia.

increase in high-molecular-weight plasma proteins there is an effect on the electrical charge on the surface of the red cells and the cells sediment rapidly and form into stacks, like a pile of coins. These stacks are referred to as **rouleaux** (Fig. 2.4) and the film is said to show increased rouleaux formation. The other abnormality of cell distribution is **red cell agglutination**. This is caused by an antibody against a red cell antigen. The antibody-coated red cells become sticky and form into irregularly shaped

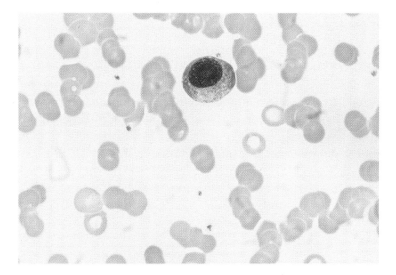

Fig. 2.4 Rouleaux.

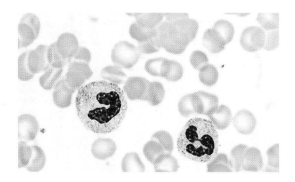

Fig. 2.5 Red cell agglutinates.

clumps or agglutinates (Fig. 2.5). Agglutinates can be distinguished from rouleaux because the clumps are an irregular jumble rather than an orderly stack. Red cell agglutinates are most often caused by an antibody which is active below normal body temperature, referred to as a cold antibody or cold agglutinin. Agglutinates will be less numerous if another film is made after the blood has been warmed. The presence of cold agglutinins can lead to anomalous blood count results.

Assessing red cell size (microcytosis, macrocytosis, anisocytosis)

Red cells are smaller than normal lymphocytes and significantly smaller than granulocytes. If cells are smaller than normal they are described as **microcytic** and if larger than normal as **macrocytic**. They are referred to as **microcytes** or **macrocytes** respectively. Red cells of normal size are said to be **normocytic**. If red cells show greater variation in size than normal the blood film is said to show **anisocytosis** (Fig. 2.6). Anisocytosis can be graded as +, ++ or +++ (mild, moderate or severe). The different sizes of red cells can be appreciated by comparing Figs 2.7, 2.8 and 2.9.

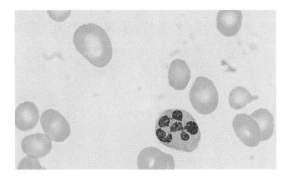

Fig. 2.6 Severe anisocytosis; the MCV was 133 fl but the macrocytosis is not uniform.

Assessing red cell shape (poikilocytosis)

If red cells show more than the normal degree of variation in red cell shape there is said to be **poikilocytosis** (Fig. 2.10).

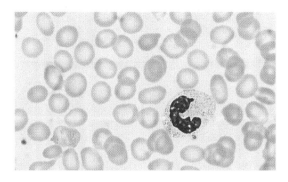

Fig. 2.7 Microcytic red cells (MCV 62 fl).

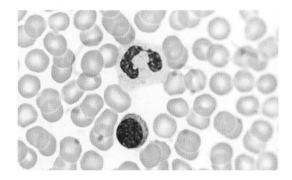

Fig. 2.8 Normocytic red cells.

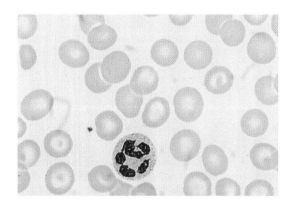

Fig. 2.9 Macrocytic red cells (MCV 105 fl).

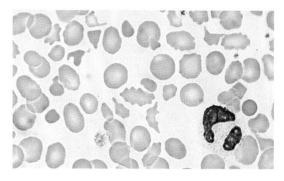

Fig. 2.10 Severe poikilocytosis; cells vary considerably in shape but no single shape dominates. (This was a case of transient severe poikilocytosis in the neonatal period in a baby with hereditary elliptocytosis.)

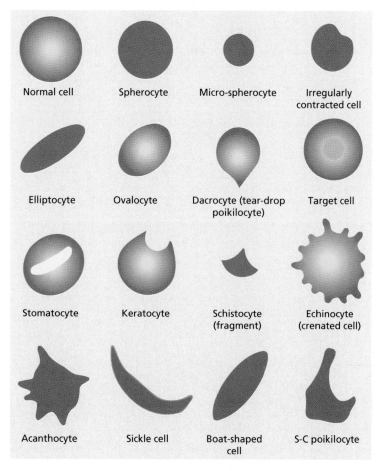

Normal cell

Spherocyte

Micro-spherocyte

Irregularly contracted cell

Elliptocyte

Ovalocyte

Dacrocyte (tear-drop poikilocyte)

Target cell

Stomatocyte

Keratocyte

Schistocyte (fragment)

Echinocyte (crenated cell)

Acanthocyte

Sickle cell

Boat-shaped cell

S-C poikilocyte

Fig. 2.11 Diagrammatic representation of different types of poikilocyte.

Individual cells of abnormal shape are referred to as **poikilocytes**. Poikilocytosis can be graded in a similar manner to anisocytosis. Individual cells of a particular shape have names which identify them, as defined in Table 2.1 and illustrated in Fig. 2.11 and Figs 2.12–2.22.

Table 2.1 Definitions of cells by shape.

Spherocyte	Cell which is approximately spherical in shape so that it has lost its central pallor; the cell outline is regular
Microspherocyte	Spherocyte of reduced size and therefore diameter
Irregularly contracted cell	Cell of reduced size and diameter with a lack of central pallor but with an irregular outline
Elliptocyte	Cell with an elliptical outline
Ovalocyte	Cell with an oval outline
Dacrocyte (tear-drop poikilocyte)	Cell shaped like a tear-drop
Target cell	Cell with a more strongly staining area in the centre of the area of central pallor
Stomatocyte	Cell with a central slit or stoma
Keratocyte	Cell with two or four curved horn-shaped projections
Schistocyte (red cell fragment)	Fragment of a cell, usually angular; a microspherocyte is a particular type of schistocyte
Echinocyte (crenated cell)	Cell with its surface covered with 20–30 small, regular, blunt projections
Acanthocyte	Cell with its surface covered with two to twenty projections of irregular shape and irregularly distributed
Sickle cell	Cell with a sickle or crescent shape, caused by the presence of a high concentration of an abnormal haemoglobin known as haemoglobin S
Boat-shaped cell	Cell similar in shape to an elliptocyte but with both ends pointed, usually indicative of the presence of haemoglobin S
SC poikilocyte	Bizarre poikilocyte formed when cells contain both haemoglobin S and haemoglobin C, having some curved edges and some square or rectangular protrusions

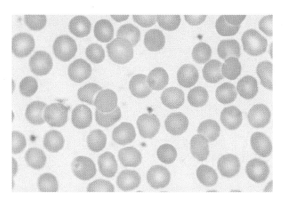

Fig. 2.12 Moderate numbers of spherocytes (in hereditary spherocytosis).

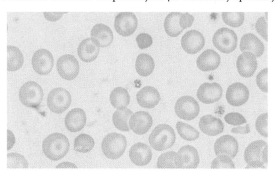

Fig. 2.13 Several irregularly contracted cells (in haemoglobin C disease). The majority of the other cells are target cells.

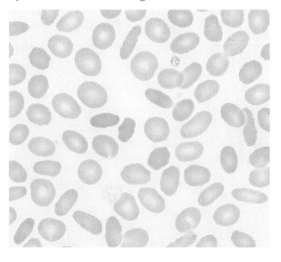

Fig. 2.14 Numerous elliptocytes and ovalocytes (in hereditary elliptocytosis).

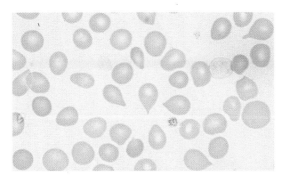

Fig. 2.15 Several dacrocytes (tear-drop poikilocytes) (in idiopathic myelofibrosis).

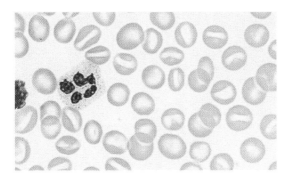

Fig. 2.16 Numerous stomatocytes (in hereditary stomatocytosis).

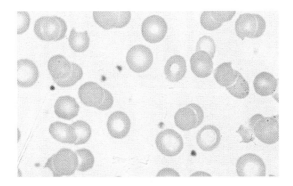

Fig. 2.17 Several keratocytes (in microangiopathic haemolytic anaemia); keratocytes are sometimes called 'bite cells' because they look as if a bite has been taken from them.

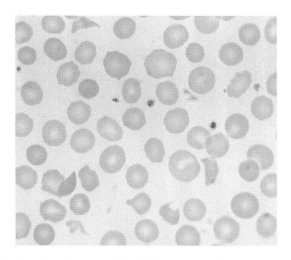

Fig. 2.18 Several schistocytes (red cell fragments) including a microspherocyte (in haemolytic uraemic syndrome).

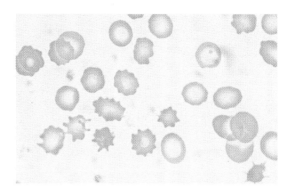

Fig. 2.19 Echinocytes (crenated cells) (in chronic renal failure).

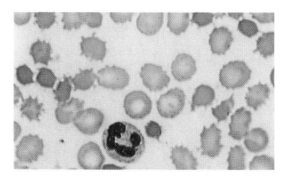

Fig. 2.20 Acanthocytes (in abetalipoproteinaemia).

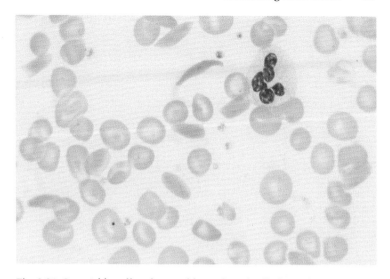

Fig. 2.21 One sickle cell and several boat-shaped cells (in sickle cell anaemia).

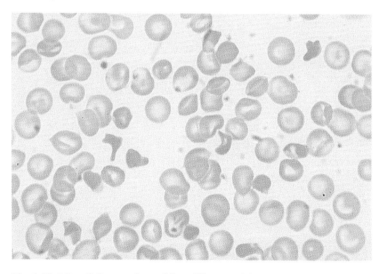

Fig. 2.22 SC poikilocytes (in sickle cell/haemoglobin C disease).

Assessing red cell colour (hypochromia, hyperchromia, anisochromasia, polychromasia)

Normal red cells are reddish-brown with approximately the central third to quarter of the cell being paler. They are described as

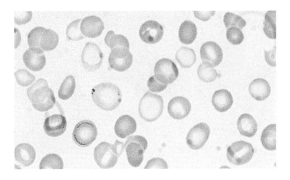

Fig. 2.23 A population of severely hypochromic cells with only a thin rim of haemoglobinized cytoplasm (in refractory anaemia with ring sideroblasts); there are other cells which stain normally and the film is therefore described as dimorphic. In addition one cell just left of centre has small basophilic inclusions, known as Pappenheimer bodies, towards the periphery of the cell.

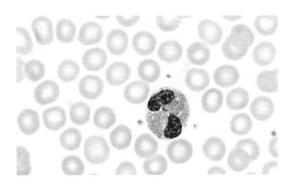

Fig. 2.24 Normochromic cells (in a healthy subject).

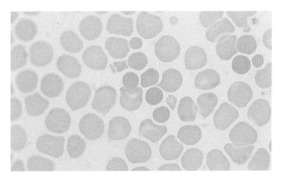

Fig. 2.25 Hyperchromic cells (which in this case are microspherocytes in a severely burned patient; spherocytes and irregularly contracted cells are also hyperchromic).

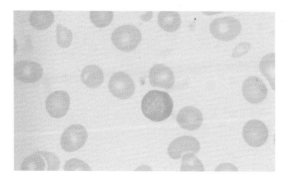

Fig. 2.26 A polychromatic macrocyte.

normochromic. Cells which have an area of central pallor more than a third of the diameter of the cell are said to be **hypochromic** and the film is said to show **hypochromia**. Cells which lack central pallor are said to be **hyperchromic**. Hypochromic, normochromic and hyperchromic cells are compared in Figs 2.23–2.25. These staining characteristics are determined by the concentration of haemoglobin in the cell and by the shape of the cell. Cells which show a greater than normal variation in the degree of haemoglobinization are said to show **anisochromasia** (see Fig. 2.1). Red cells which have a blue or lilac tinge are said to show **polychromasia** ('many colours'). **Polychromatic cells** (Fig. 2.26) are young cells, newly released from the bone marrow. They have not yet been remodelled to the disc shape of a mature erythrocyte and therefore lack central pallor. They are also generally larger than more mature cells and in this case may be described as **polychromatic macrocytes**. Young red cells can also be detected with a special stain of live (unfixed) cells called a supravital stain. Young cells detected in this way are called **reticulocytes** because the supravital staining causes a network or 'reticulum' to be deposited. Another word usually used to describe staining characteristics of red cells is **dimorphic**. The word means that there are two types of cell but it is most often applied to a mixture of hypochromic and normochromic cells (see Fig. 2.23). The two populations of cells usually differ in size as well as in staining characteristics. A dimorphic film differs from

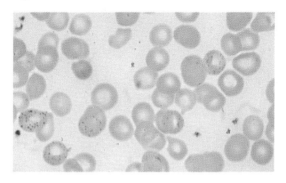

Fig. 2.27 Numerous cells showing basophilic stippling (in lead poisoning). Punctate basophilia is an alternative term used to describe this abnormality.

one showing anisochromasia in that there are two distinct populations of cells rather than a gradation of staining characteristics.

Detecting red cell inclusions (Pappenheimer bodies, basophilic stippling, Howell–Jolly bodies)

Red cells may contain inclusions. **Pappenheimer bodies** are small, basophilic inclusions, occurring in small numbers towards the periphery of the cell (see Fig. 2.23). They contain iron and when this is confirmed by an iron stain they are referred to as siderotic granules. **Basophilic stippling** refers to the presence of small basophilic inclusions distributed throughout the red cell (Fig. 2.27). They do not contain iron but represent abnormally staining ribosomes. **Howell–Jolly bodies** (Fig. 2.28) are larger, round, densely staining inclusions, usually towards one edge of the cell. They represent a nuclear fragment that was not extruded when the red cell left the bone marrow. Usually any Howell–Jolly bodies left in red cells as they leave the bone marrow are removed by the spleen. They are therefore most often seen in people who have had their spleens removed.

Malaria parasites are intracellular and are detected as inclusions within red cells. Their detection is very important in diag-

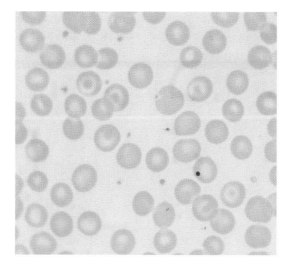

Fig. 2.28 A cell containing a Howell–Jolly body in a patient who has had a splenectomy. There are also several target cells.

nosis and as yet there is no reliable substitute for the blood film in their detection.

The full blood count in red cell assessment

The blood count is very important in detecting or confirming the presence of anaemia, polycythaemia, microcytosis and macrocytosis. Some instruments also detect hypochromia and hyperchromia by changes in the MCHC. Most instruments can detect the presence of two cell populations which would produce a dimorphic blood film. Many instruments also produce a measurement called the **red cell distribution width (RDW)**, which quantitates anisocytosis. Some also produce a measurement called the **haemoglobin distribution width (HDW)**, which is indicative of the degree of anisochromasia.

The adequate assessment of an abnormal blood count often requires the examination of a blood film since there are many abnormalities detectable on blood films which are not detected by automated counters, e.g. the presence of poikilocytes, red cell inclusions or increased rouleaux formation. The presence of red cell agglutinates can sometimes be suspected because of very abnormal and improbable FBC results but a blood film is needed for confirmation.

CHAPTER 3

Assessing White Cells and Platelets

White cells and platelets may be increased or decreased in number. They may also show morphological abnormalities, either inherited or acquired. Assessing whether the numbers of individual types of white cell are increased or decreased requires a differential count. However, the differential count is of little importance in itself and should only be used to calculate the absolute numbers of each cell type. The absolute counts are then compared with those expected in healthy people of the same age, sex and ethnic group. The terms used in describing numerical abnormalities in white cells and platelets are defined in Table 3.1.

Table 3.1 Terminology used for abnormalities of white cell and platelet numbers.

Leucocytosis	Increased white cell count
Neutrophilia (or neutrophil leucocytosis)	Increased neutrophil count
Lymphocytosis	Increased lymphocyte count
Monocytosis	Increased monocyte count
Eosinophilia	Increased eosinophil count
Basophilia	Increased basophil count
Thrombocytosis	Increased platelet count
Leucopenia	Decreased white cell count
Neutropenia	Decreased neutrophil count
Lymphopenia (or lymphocytopenia)	Decreased lymphocyte count
Monocytopenia	Decreased monocyte count
Eosinopenia	Decreased eosinophil count
Basopenia	Decreased basophil count
Thrombocytopenia	Decreased platelet count

Assessing white cell and platelet numbers

White blood cell counts can be assessed by examining a blood film, preferably by low power, but an instrumental WBC is much more precise. Figure 3.1 illustrates leucocytosis. In comparison, if the WBC were normal, no more than one or two cells would be expected in a microscopic field of this size and if there were leucopenia many such fields would contain no white cells.

Platelet numbers can also be assessed on a film, by relating their number to the number of red cells present. An instrument platelet count is generally much more precise than an estimate from a film but is prone to errors because of poor specimen collection techniques or characteristics of the sample. If a platelet count is unexpectedly low it is important to check that this is not because the specimen is partially clotted. Some automated instruments have a mechanism for checking for clots but otherwise this has to be done manually by the laboratory worker. It is important that all low platelet counts are confirmed on a blood film. Figures 3.1, 3.2 and 3.3 contrast normal, high and low platelet counts. It is also important to examine a blood film in all cases with apparent thrombocytopenia to exclude platelet aggregation or satellitism (see Figs 1.21 & 1.23) as a cause of a falsely low count.

Assessing neutrophil morphology

Neutrophils may show increased (Fig. 3.4) or decreased (see Fig. 1.13) granulation. Increased granulation is usually a reaction to infection or inflammation and is therefore referred to as **toxic granulation**. However, it does also occur as a normal phenomenon, during pregnancy. Cytoplasmic inclusions may be present as an inherited or acquired abnormality. The commonest such abnormality is a small, pale, blue–grey inclusion which occurs both during pregnancy and in infection and inflammation and is known as a **Döhle body** (Fig. 3.5). Another common cytoplasmic abnormality, which is strongly suggestive of infection, is cytoplasmic vacuolation (Fig. 3.4).

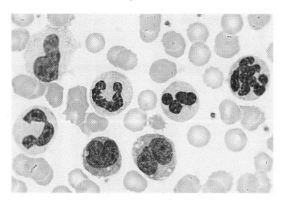

Fig. 3.1 Leucocytosis.

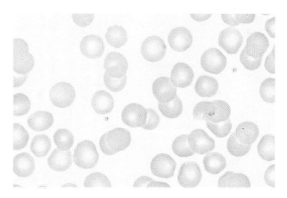

Fig. 3.2 Thrombocytopenia (in Wiskott–Aldrich syndrome). There are only two platelets in the film. The platelets are also abnormally small, although their staining characteristics are normal.

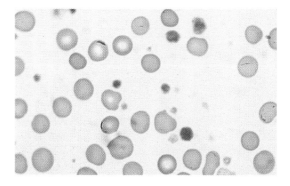

Fig. 3.3 Thrombocytosis (in chronic granulocytic leukaemia). The platelets also show increased variation in size and some are agranular.

Neutrophils may have congenital or acquired abnormalities of nuclear lobulation. An increase in band forms and less lobulated neutrophils in relation to more mature, well-lobulated neutrophils is known as a **left shift** (Fig. 3.4). This term is also used when neutrophil precursors are present in the blood. Neutrophils

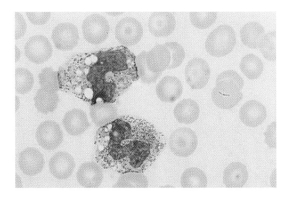

Fig. 3.4 Toxic granulation, vacuolation and left shift (the two white cells are band forms).

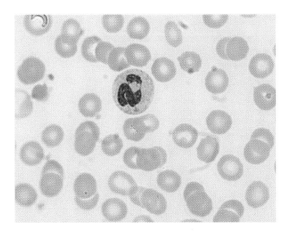

Fig. 3.5 A neutrophil containing a Döhle body, a small blue–grey cytoplasmic inclusion which can be seen just below the nucleus.

may also be hypolobulated, but with very round lobes and with some nuclei being shaped like a pair of spectacles or a peanut. This occurs as a congenital abnormality known as the Pelger–Huët anomaly (Fig. 3.6). There will be some neutrophils with completely round nuclei. This congenital anomaly is of no clinical significance but it is important not to confuse it with left shift. A similar abnormality can develop as an acquired condition known as the pseudo- or acquired Pelger–Huët anomaly. The acquired Pelger–Huët anomaly is clinically very significant because it is a feature of a neoplastic condition, called a myelodysplastic syndrome, which may lead on to acute leukaemia. The nuclei have similar abnormal shapes in the congenital and acquired Pelger–Huët anomalies but in the latter there are often associated abnormalities (e.g. neutropenia or hypogranular neutrophils). Neutrophils may also show increased lobulation (Fig. 3.7). This is known as **right shift**. Neutrophils with six or more lobes are said to be hypersegmented. **Neutrophil hypersegmentation** is an important clue to the presence of deficiency of vitamin B_{12} or folic acid. **Macropolycytes** (Fig. 3.8) should not be confused with hypersegmented neutrophils: they are twice the size of normal neutrophils and the nucleus is twice as big. This is because one cell division has been missed during neutrophil production. Macropolycytes are likely to have 92

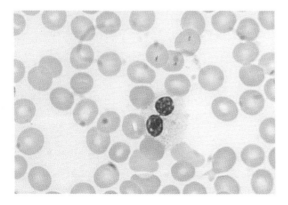

Fig. 3.6 A neutrophil with two very round lobes in a patient with the congenital Pelger–Huët anomaly.

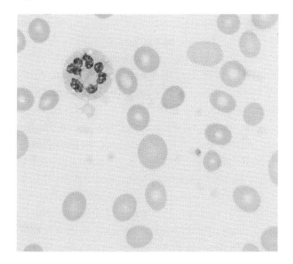

Fig. 3.7 A hypersegmented neutrophil in a patient with megaloblastic anaemia. The neutrophil nucleus has seven lobes.

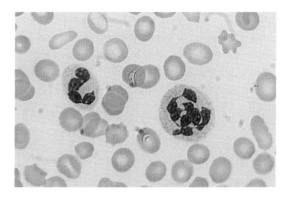

Fig. 3.8 A macropolycyte compared with a normal neutrophil. The macropolycyte is twice as large as the normal neutrophil and has a nucleus with seven or eight lobes which is also twice as large as a normal neutrophil nucleus.

rather than 46 chromosomes, i.e. they are likely to be tetraploid rather than diploid. Although their nuclei may have six or more lobes, macropolycytes do not have the same significance as hypersegmented neutrophils and should be distinguished from them.

Granulocyte precursors and nucleated red cells may be present simultaneously in the peripheral blood. This can occur as a normal phenomenon in pregnancy but otherwise it is mainly seen in severely ill patients, who are usually anaemic. The anaemia is referred to as a **leucoerythroblastic anaemia**. Leucoerythroblastic anaemia is indicative of either a bone marrow disease (e.g. idiopathic myelofibrosis), bone marrow infiltration (e.g. by carcinoma cells) or a severe systemic illness (e.g. severe infection or haemorrhagic shock).

Assessing lymphocyte morphology

Congenital abnormalities of lymphocytes are rare. Most abnormalities of lymphocyte morphology are caused by viral infections. Less often, increased numbers of lymphocytes showing a variable degree of morphological abnormality are indicative of a neoplastic process, either a lymphoid leukaemia or a lymphoma (see Chapter 4). The most striking reactive changes in lymphocyte morphology are seen in infectious mononucleosis, an illness caused by an acute infection by the Epstein–Barr (EB) virus. There is lymphocytosis and lymphocytes are morphologically very abnormal (Fig. 3.9). Some are very large, some have primitive nuclei with a diffuse chromatin pattern and nucleoli, some nuclei are lobulated, some cells have voluminous basophilic cytoplasm. The cells are pleomorphic, i.e. they vary greatly in size and shape. The lymphocytes are so abnormal that initially their true nature was not known and they were referred to as **atypical mononuclear cells**. Now they are more often referred to as **atypical lymphocytes**. Large numbers of atypical lymphocytes, similar to those seen in infectious mononucleosis, can also occur in infection by cytomegalovirus, hepatitis A virus and adenovirus and during the parasitic infection, toxoplasmosis. Smaller numbers of atypical lymphocytes are seen in many other viral, bacterial, rickettsial and protozoan infections.

Other reactive changes, in addition to those typical of infectious mononucleosis, occur in lymphocytes both during infection and during exposure to other antigenic stimuli. B lymphocytes may differentiate into plasma cells (Fig. 3.10) with an increased amount of basophilic cytoplasm, a pale-staining

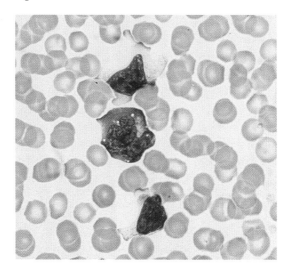

Fig. 3.9 Atypical lymphocytes (in infectious mononucleosis).

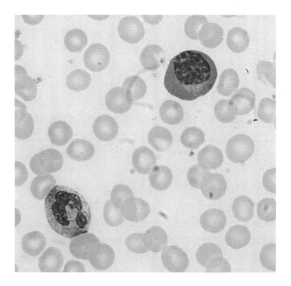

Fig. 3.10 A plasma cell (occurring as a reactive change in a patient with infection). The chromatin is clumped and a Golgi zone is apparent below the nucleus.

area near the nucleus (the Golgi zone) and an eccentric nucleus with clumped chromatin. There may also be plasmacytoid lymphocytes with characteristics intermediate between those of lymphocytes and plasma cells. An increase of large granular lymphocytes can also occur as a reactive change, e.g. during chronic viral infection. These cells may be indistinguishable from normal large granular lymphocytes but sometimes they show features of activation such as a larger size and more voluminous basophilic cytoplasm.

Characteristic morphological changes occur in lymphocytes in different types of leukaemia and lymphoma (see Chapter 4).

Assessing morphology of monocytes, eosinophils and basophils

Numerical changes in monocytes, eosinophils and basophils are often useful in diagnosis but this is less often the case with morphological changes.

Monocytes can show increased size and cytoplasmic vacuolation during infection. Immature monocytes with increased gran-

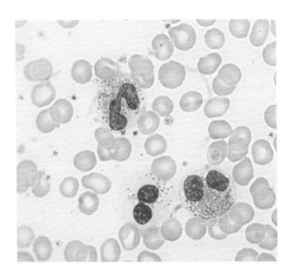

Fig. 3.11 Eosinophil leucocytosis with one of the three eosinophils being markedly hypogranular.

ulation and cytoplasmic basophilia can occur both in infections and in leukaemia and related conditions.

Eosinophils can show a variety of morphological abnormalities (Fig. 3.11) including hyper- and hypolobulation, reduced granulation and cytoplasmic vacuolation. However, these changes occur in reactive eosinophilia (e.g. in parasitic infection) and also in eosinophilic leukaemia so they are not useful in differential diagnosis.

Basophils sometimes show reduced granulation but since this can occur as a laboratory artefact as well as during allergic reactions and in leukaemia and related disorders, its detection is not very helpful in diagnosis.

Assessing platelet morphology

Platelets may be smaller than normal (Fig. 3.2) or, more often, larger than normal (Fig. 3.3). Very large platelets are sometimes referred to as giant platelets. An increased variability in platelet size is referred to as platelet anisocytosis (Fig. 3.3). Platelet size is of diagnostic significance, particularly if considered in relation to the platelet count. Small or normal-size platelets in association with thrombocytopenia suggest that the cause is a failure of bone marrow production, whereas thrombocytopenia with large platelets is more likely to be caused by peripheral destruction or consumption of platelets with the bone marrow responding by increasing platelet production. Platelet size is also useful in assessing the likely cause of thrombocytosis. In reactive thrombocytosis (e.g. caused by severe infection or inflammation) the platelets are usually of normal size, whereas when thrombocytosis is a feature of a myeloproliferative disorder (chronic granulocytic leukaemia, essential thrombocythaemia or polycythaemia rubra vera) platelet size is generally increased and some giant platelets are present.

Platelets may show defective or absent granulation. Often this is an artefactual change, because the blood specimen has partly clotted or because platelets have aggregated and have discharged some or all of their granules (see Fig. 1.21). If an artefact is excluded then the detection of defectively granulated platelets is of diagnostic significance. It occurs as a rare congenital anomaly (the grey platelet syndrome), but usually it is consequent on a bone marrow disease such as one of the myeloproliferative or myelodysplastic disorders.

CHAPTER 4

Haematological Findings in Health and Disease

The blood film and count in healthy individuals

The microscopic features of normal blood cells and the normal range for the blood count have been discussed in Chapter 1. In assessing what is 'normal' it is necessary to consider the gender, age and ethnic origin of the person being investigated.

Gender

Adult men have a higher normal range for RBC, Hb and PCV/Hct than adult women but women tend to have a somewhat higher WBC and platelet count (see Table 1.2).

Neonates, infants, and children

The blood counts of healthy neonates, infants and children differ greatly from those of healthy adults (see Table 1.3). Neonates have a higher Hb, MCV, WBC, neutrophil count and lymphocyte count than adults. Children in general have a higher lymphocyte count than adults. They tend to have a slightly lower Hb and MCV.

Pregnancy

Physiological variation in the blood count occurs during pregnancy. The Hb falls, the MCV rises slightly and the WBC and neutrophil count rise. Immature cells (myelocytes and occasional promyelocytes) appear in the blood and there may be 'toxic' granulation and Döhle bodies.

Ethnic variation

The blood counts of healthy Africans and Afro-Caribbeans (see Table 1.3) often show a lower white cell and neutrophil count than is usual in Caucasians (see Table 1.2). There is also a tendency to a lower platelet count, particularly in Africans.

Abnormalities of red cells

Polycythaemia

Polycythaemia is an increase in the Hb. It is usually accompanied by an increase in the RBC and PCV/Hct. It can be caused by a true increase in the total volume of red cells in the circulation (true polycythaemia) or by a decrease in the total plasma volume (apparent or relative or pseudo-polycythaemia). It is not possible to distinguish true from apparent polycythaemia by a blood film or count. True polycythaemia is caused by overproduction of red cells. Normally red cell production is driven by erythropoietin production in response to a diminished oxygen supply to the kidney. Overproduction of red cells may be an erythropoietin-mediated physiological response to hypoxia or it may be caused by inappropriate secretion of erythropoietin or by mechanisms independent of erythropoietin. Some of the important causes of polycythaemia, classified according to mechanism, are shown in Table 4.1.

Polycythaemia vera

Polycythaemia vera, also referred to as polycythaemia rubra vera or primary proliferative polycythaemia, is a myeloproliferative disorder characterized by overproduction of red cells. In many patients there is also overproduction of white cells and platelets. Clinical features are facial plethora and sometimes a moderate degree of splenomegaly. The disease may be complicated by arterial thrombosis and peripheral ischaemia.

Table 4.1 Some important causes of polycythaemia, classified according to mechanism.

Relative polycythaemia	Acute loss of water from the body or plasma from the blood stream, e.g. dehydration, shock or burns
	Chronic reduction of plasma volume, sometimes due to cigarette smoking, sometimes idiopathic, diuretic use
True polycythaemia, erythropoietin-mediated, resulting from hypoxia	Living at a high altitude, hypoxic lung disease, cyanotic heart disease, hypoventilation (e.g. due to extreme obesity)
True polycythaemia, erythropoietin-mediated, resulting from tissue hypoxia	High-affinity haemoglobin or abnormal haemoglobin without oxygen-carrying capacity, e.g. increased carboxyhaemoglobin in heavy smokers or methaemoglobinaemia (congenital or acquired)
True polycythaemia, erythropoietin-mediated, due to inadequate blood supply to the kidney	Renal artery stenosis
True polycythaemia due to inappropriate erythropoietin secretion	Renal disease: renal cysts, renal tumours
	Other inappropriate erythropoietin production: hepatic tumours, cerebellar haemangioblastoma, uterine fibroids
True polycythaemia, independent of erythropoietin, due to intrinsic bone marrow disease	Polycythaemia vera

The blood film is 'packed'. The number of neutrophils, basophils, and platelets may be increased and some giant platelets may be present. Increased numbers of basophils are particularly important in diagnosis since they are not increased in any of the other causes of true or apparent polycythaemia.

Further steps: Confirm the high Hb on a repeat blood sample. Check history and physical findings. Is the patient hypoxic or a heavy smoker? Check the blood film for neutrophilia, basophilia and giant platelets. If the cause is not obvious, measure red cell mass and plasma volume to check if this is a true or a relative polycythaemia. If it is a true polycythaemia and the patient is not hypoxic, do an ultrasound examination of the abdomen to assess the kidneys and spleen, measure serum erythropoietin concentration and do a trephine biopsy of the bone marrow.

Anaemia and other disorders of red cell production

Anaemia is a reduction of the Hb, usually accompanied by a reduction in the RBC and PCV/Hct. A reduction of the RBC, Hb and PCV/Hct can also be factitious, when a blood specimen has been taken from a vein above an intravenous infusion or when there has been poor mixing of the specimen in the laboratory. Laboratory workers must be alert to the possibility of such misleading results. Table 4.2 summarizes the causes of anaemia, according to mechanism. Anaemia can also be classified according to cell size, as microcytic, normocytic or macrocytic. This is useful as it directs investigation to a more limited range of

Table 4.2 Some important causes of anaemia, classified according to mechanism.

Blood loss
Reduced red cell life span (haemolytic anaemia)
 Consequent on an intrinsic abnormality of red cells, either inherited
  (e.g. hereditary spherocytosis or haemoglobin C disease) or acquired
  (e.g. paroxysmal nocturnal haemoglobinuria)
 Consequent on extrinsic (vascular or plasma) factors (e.g. haemolytic
  uraemic syndrome, autoimmune haemolytic anaemia)
Inadequate production of red cells
 Deficiency or iron, vitamin B_{12} or folic acid
 Aplastic or hypoplastic anaemias, either inherited or acquired (e.g.
  Fanconi's anaemia or drug-induced aplastic anaemia)
 Ineffective production of red cells (e.g. myelodysplastic syndromes)
 Bone marrow infiltration by malignant cells
 Bone marrow fibrosis
*Low-affinity haemoglobin**
Abnormal distribution of red cells within the vasculature
 Hypersplenism

*A rare mechanism of anaemia except that this is one of the causes of the low Hb in sickle cell anaemia.

Table 4.3 Some causes of anaemia with microcytic, normocytic or macrocytic red cells.

Causes of microcytic anaemia
    Iron deficiency anaemia
    Anaemia of chronic disease
    Thalassaemia (but thalassaemia trait more often causes microcytosis
        without anaemia)
    Congenital sideroblastic anaemia

Causes of normocytic anaemia
    Early iron deficiency anaemia
    Early anaemia of chronic disease
    Recent blood loss
    Combined deficiency of iron and either folic acid or vitamin B_{12}
    Renal failure
    Haemolytic anaemia (but may also be macrocytic)

Causes of macrocytic anaemia
    Vitamin B_{12} deficiency
    Folic acid deficiency
    Administration of certain drugs (e.g. hydroxyurea, azathioprine,
        zidovudine)
    Liver disease
    Alcohol excess
    Hypothyroidism
    Haemolytic anaemia
    Myelodysplastic syndromes

possibilities (Table 4.3). Anaemia can also be classified according to the appearance of the red cells, e.g. as a spherocytic anaemia or as a microangiopathic haemolytic anaemia. The more important causes of anaemia will be discussed, together with other disorders of red cell production, in the following pages.

Megaloblastic anaemia

Megaloblastic anaemia usually results from a deficiency of either vitamin B_{12} or folic acid. It can occur at any age but is commonest in the elderly. Clinical features are those of anaemia (e.g. pallor, fatigue, breathlessness) and in addition there may be mild jaundice, inflammation of the tongue (glossitis) and, in the case of vitamin B_{12} deficiency, neurological complications.

The diagnosis can only be made with certainty from a bone marrow examination, which shows asynchrony between nuclear and cytoplasmic maturation, nuclear maturation being retarded. However, the blood film and count are often so typical that there is little doubt as to the diagnosis and, if further investigations can be done rapidly and provide a definitive diagnosis, bone marrow examination is not necessary.

The blood film (see Fig. 3.7) shows anaemia, macrocytosis, anisocytosis and poikilocytosis. Macrocytes include both round and oval macrocytes (whereas round macrocytes alone are characteristic of macrocytosis for other reasons, e.g. liver disease or ethanol excess). Anisocytosis and poikilocytosis become marked as the anaemia becomes more severe. Poikilocytes include oval cells, teardrop poikilocytes and red cell fragments. When anaemia is severe, there may be some circulating NRBC, which show the nucleocytoplasmic asynchrony of megaloblastic erythropoiesis (Fig. 4.1). Neutrophils are hypersegmented; there is an increase in the mean lobe count, the proportion of five-lobed neutrophils is increased and some neutrophils with six, seven or more lobes may be present. There may also be a few macropolycytes.

The FBC shows a fall in the Hb and PCV/Hct and a parallel increase in the MCV and MCH. Mean cell haemoglobin concentration is normal. There is a marked fall in the RBC. The RDW is increased. When anaemia is very severe the rise in the MCV is not as marked as might be expected. This is because of the

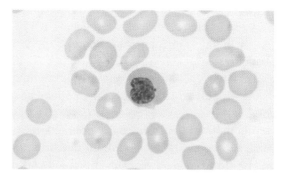

Fig. 4.1 Megaloblastic anaemia showing macrocytosis and a circulating megaloblast.

concomitant marked anisocytosis and poikilocytosis with many red cell fragments and small poikilocytes. With severe anaemia the RDW is very abnormal and the HDW is also increased. In severe cases the WBC and platelet count are reduced.

Further steps: Check clinical history and physical findings. Is the diet deficient in vitamin B_{12} (vegan or very restricted vegetarian diet) or folic acid (lack of liver and fresh fruit and vegetables)? Has the patient had a total gastrectomy? Do the history or the physical findings suggest alcohol excess, liver disease or malabsorption? Is the patient taking a drug known to cause macrocytosis? Are there neurological features suggestive of vitamin B_{12} deficiency (peripheral neuropathy, optic neuropathy, subacute combined degeneration of the spinal cord, dementia)?

Assay serum vitamin B_{12} and red cell folate and do liver and thyroid function tests. Consider whether a bone marrow aspirate is needed. If vitamin B_{12} concentration is reduced, test for antibodies to gastric parietal cells and intrinsic factor and consider a Schilling test. If coeliac disease is suspected, test for antibodies to endomysium and gliadin.

If haemolytic anaemia is possible, examine blood film for polychromasia and specific features of various haemolytic anaemias, do reticulocyte count and measure serum bilirubin and lactate dehydrogenase.

Iron deficiency anaemia

Iron deficiency anaemia occurs when the body's stores of iron are insufficient to maintain erythropoiesis. It occurs at any age but is commonest in infancy, in menstruating girls and women and during pregnancy. Clinical features are those of anaemia. Severe cases may also have cracking at the corners of the mouth (angular cheilosis), atrophic glossitis and flat or spoon-shaped nails (koilonychia).

The anaemia that develops is initially normocytic and normochromic and subsequently hypochromic and microcytic (Fig. 4.2). There is mild to moderate anisocytosis and poikilocytosis. Poikilocytes often include elliptocytes. The long, thin elliptocytes of iron deficiency are sometimes referred to as pencil cells.

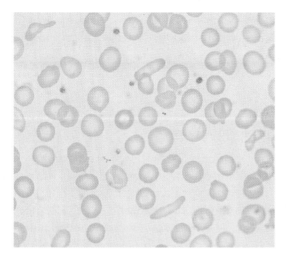

Fig. 4.2 Iron deficiency anaemia showing anisocytosis, anisochromasia and the presence of poikilocytes including elliptocytes (pencil cells).

Target cells are uncommon and anisochromasia is characteristic, two features that can be useful in making the distinction from thalassaemia trait. The platelet count is sometimes increased.

The FBC initially shows a fall in the Hb and a rise in the RDW. Subsequently there is a fall in the MCV and the MCH and, when it is measured by a sensitive technique, a fall in the MCHC.

Further steps: Check history and physical findings. Is the diet adequate (vegetarian diets are often deficient in iron)? Is the patient a rapidly growing child or adolescent or a woman who has had repeated pregnancies? Is there a history of blood loss, e.g. heavy menses (menorrhagia), vomiting blood (haematemesis), passing black stools (melaena—indicative of upper gastrointestinal blood loss)? Does the patient take aspirin or other drugs that cause gastric ulceration or have a history of indigestion or difficulty swallowing? Is there any bowel dysfunction suggestive of malabsorption or a bowel lesion that could cause occult haemorrhage? Consider testing for coeliac disease (antiendomysial and antigliadin antibodies).

Measure serum ferritin (low level confirms iron deficiency) or *both* serum iron *and* iron-binding capacity or transferrin concentration (a low serum iron does not confirm iron deficiency unless it is accompanied by a raised iron-binding capacity/ transferrin).

Remember, it is not sufficient to merely confirm a diagnosis of iron deficiency. You must also find the reason.

Anaemia of chronic disease

The anaemia of chronic disease (Fig. 4.3) can result from chronic infection, from chronic inflammatory diseases such as rheumatoid arthritis, or from malignant disease. Clinical features are those of anaemia and of the primary disease. The mechanism of anaemia is reduced delivery of iron from the reticuloendothelial system to the developing erythroblast together with a blunted erythropoietin response to anaemia and a minor degree of shortening of red cell survival. The anaemia is initially normocytic and normochromic, but, when the condition is chronic and severe, hypochromia and microcytosis may be marked. Poikilocytosis is not marked. Because of an increased concentration of plasma proteins, rouleaux formation is usually more marked than in iron deficiency anaemia of equivalent severity and the erythrocyte sedimentation rate (ESR) shows a more marked increase. Other signs of an inflammatory response such as increased background staining, neutrophilia and thrombocytosis occur if the underlying disease is severe.

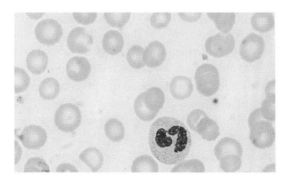

Fig. 4.3 Anaemia of chronic disease showing microcytosis, hypochromia and anisochromasia.

It may be impossible to distinguish between iron deficiency anaemia and the anaemia of chronic disease on the basis of the blood count and film, and assessment of iron stores is then needed.

Further steps: Check the history and physical findings. Is there evidence of infection, an inflammatory condition or a malignant disease? Are there laboratory markers of inflammation such as neutrophilia, an increased ESR, increased C-reactive protein, increased serum globulins. Measure ferritin (normal or high) or *both* serum iron *and* iron-binding capacity or transferrin (all low). If it is not clear whether the patient has iron deficiency or the anaemia of chronic disease or a combination of the two, consider a bone marrow aspirate to assess iron stores.

Beta thalassaemia trait

Beta thalassaemia trait is the abnormality resulting from reduced or absent function of one of the two beta globin genes. The individual is heterozygous for a beta thalassaemia gene, β^0 or β^+ thalassaemia. The condition occurs in many ethnic groups including populations from around the Mediterranean and from the Indian sub-continent and South-East Asia, Africans, Afro-Caribbean and Arabs. This is usually an asymptomatic condition, but, since the offspring of two carriers of beta thalassaemia trait may suffer from thalassaemia major, its detection is important. The diagnosis is most readily suspected from the FBC. The Hb is usually normal or only slightly reduced although it may be lower during pregnancy or intercurrent infection. The MCV and MCH are reduced and the RBC is elevated. The MCHC may be slightly reduced when it is measured by a sensitive instrument. The high RBC is useful in making a distinction from iron deficiency since a high RBC is quite uncommon in iron deficiency. The RDW is more often normal in thalassaemia trait than in iron deficiency.

The blood film may show only microcytosis and in such cases the diagnosis may not be suspected from the blood film. In other cases (Fig. 4.4) there is also hypochromia and the presence of poikilocytes including target cells. Some patients have promi-

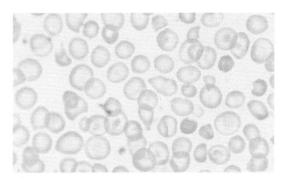

Fig. 4.4 Beta thalassaemia trait showing microcytosis, hypochromia and poikilocytosis. The poikilocytes include target cells and several irregularly contracted cells.

nent basophilic stippling and some have small numbers of irregularly contracted cells. These two features are not expected in iron deficiency and their presence is therefore useful in the differential diagnosis of microcytosis.

However, since blood film abnormalities may be subtle, diagnosis is dependent on the blood count and on carrying out a specific test (measurement of haemoglobin A$_2$ concentration) whenever a low MCV and MCH suggest the possibility of this diagnosis.

Further steps: Check the ethnic origin of the patient. Measure the haemoglobin A$_2$ percentage. A high level generally confirms beta thalassaemia trait. Don't forget that genetic counselling may be needed. If the red cell indices are typical of thalassaemia trait but the haemoglobin A$_2$ is normal, consider the possibility of alpha thalassaemia trait (see below). Less often, such indices are the result of polycythaemia that has been treated by repeated venesection and has caused iron deficiency—check the clinical history.

Alpha thalassaemia trait

Alpha thalassaemia trait is the abnormality resulting from absence or reduced function of either one or two of the four alpha globin genes. It is an asymptomatic condition. It is commonest among Africans and Afro-Caribbeans and in Chinese and South-East Asian populations. Not all cases show an abnormality of the blood film or count. Patients who lack only one of the four alpha globin genes may have mild microcytosis or may be haematologically normal. Patients who lack two alpha globin genes usually have an abnormality very similar to that of beta thalassaemia trait, although basophilic stippling and target cells are less common.

Further steps: Usually the diagnosis of alpha thalassaemia trait does not matter. However, in certain ethnic groups (Chinese, South-East Asian, Greek, Cypriot, Turkish) there may be a chromosome with no alpha genes. This is called α^0 thalassaemia and if it is present in both parents it can cause a severe anaemia, incompatible with life, in a fetus. So check the ethnic origin and arrange DNA analysis if the individual could have alpha thalassaemia trait and if this would be clinically relevant. If the MCH is 26 fl or higher, α^0 thalassaemia is very unlikely. Confirmation of the diagnosis of α^+ thalassaemia, the milder condition in which only one of the two alpha genes on a chromosome is missing, is not generally necessary.

Haemoglobin H disease

Haemoglobin H disease is an inherited condition characterized by a moderately severe anaemia attributable in part to reduced synthesis of haemoglobin and in part to haemolysis. It is caused by deletion of three of the four alpha globin genes (or by mutations of alpha globin genes leading to a similar reduction of alpha globin synthesis). The reduced alpha globin production leads to a thalassaemic disorder and to the production of an abnormal haemoglobin, haemoglobin H, which has four beta globin chains and no alpha chains. Haemoglobin H is present as a minor component, the majority of haemoglobin being haemoglobin A. Haemoglobin H disease occurs in South-East Asia and around the Mediterranean. Clinical features are anaemia and splenomegaly.

The blood film (Fig. 4.5) shows hypochromia and marked microcytosis and anisocytosis. Poikilocytosis is very striking with poikilocytes including red cell fragments, teardrop poikilocytes

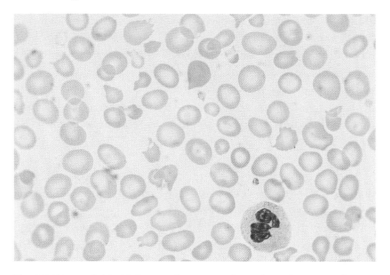

Fig. 4.5 Haemoglobin H disease showing moderate hypochromia and marked microcytosis, anisocytosis and poikilocytosis.

and target cells. There is polychromasia, correlating with an increased reticulocyte count.

The Hb is moderately reduced (usually 6–10 g/dl). There is marked reduction of the MCV and MCH, reduction of the MCHC and an increased RDW and HDW.

Further steps: Look for haemoglobin H inclusions by a specific stain and look for haemoglobin H by haemoglobin electrophoresis or high performance liquid chromatography (HPLC). Check for a raised reticulocyte count. Check the parents—at least one of them should have only two alpha genes and thus should have obvious alpha thalassaemia trait with an MCH less than 26 fl.

Hyposplenism

Reduced or absent splenic function is referred to as hyposplenism. It can result from congenital absence or surgical removal of the spleen or from loss of splenic function, e.g. because of splenic atrophy or infarction. The blood film (see Fig. 2.28) shows target cells, Howell–Jolly bodies, acanthocytes, occasional spherocytes, occasional Pappenheimer bodies and some giant platelets. The blood count may show increased neutrophils, lymphocytes or platelets.

A degree of hyposplenism is normal in the neonatal period, particularly in premature neonates. Otherwise hyposplenism is abnormal and its detection is important. Patients may be unaware that a splenectomy has been carried out in the past, and they and their physicians may therefore be unaware of the consequent risk of overwhelming infection and the need for prophylactic penicillin and certain vaccinations. Hyposplenism can also provide a diagnostic clue to conditions such as coeliac disease that can be associated with splenic atrophy.

When splenectomy is carried out in a patient with a haematological abnormality, post-splenectomy features are often modified or aggravated by the effects of the underlying disease. It is also important to note the features of hyposplenism, when present, since this might explain a haematological abnormality such as thrombocytosis or lymphocytosis and avoid unnecessary further investigations.

Further steps: Check the history. Is the patient known to have had a splenectomy or is there a history of a disease associated with splenic atrophy (coeliac disease or dermatitis herpetiformis) or replacement of functioning splenic tissue (amyloidosis)? Consider a CT scan or other imaging technique to confirm unexpected hyposplenism, as this is an important diagnosis.

Hereditary spherocytosis

The term hereditary spherocytosis covers a heterogeneous group of inherited red cell membrane disorders characterized by a membrane spectrin deficiency, spherocytic red cells and either haemolytic anaemia or compensated haemolysis. Inheritance is most often autosomal dominant. Cases occur among many ethnic groups. Clinical features can include anaemia, jaundice and the complications of gallstones.

The blood film shows that some, but not usually all, of the red cells lack central pallor (see Fig. 2.12). In patients with anaemia there may be polychromasia. The Hb may be normal or reduced.

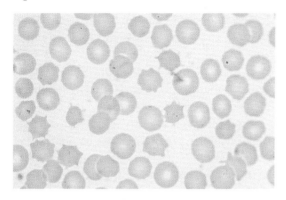

Fig. 4.6 Spherocytes, spheroacanthocytes and red cells containing Pappenheimer bodies following splenectomy for hereditary spherocytosis.

MCHC is increased when it is measured by a sensitive method. After splenectomy, spheroacanthocytes, i.e. spherical cells with irregular spicules, may be very prominent (Fig. 4.6).

Further steps: Check the family history and, if necessary, the blood counts and films of both parents. An osmotic fragility test confirms the present of spherocytes but is not necessary if it is obvious that there are spherocytes. An autoimmune haemolytic anaemia is an important differential diagnosis, so check the direct antiglobulin test (Coombs' test). If the patient is in hospital, check that there has not been a recent blood transfusion since a delayed haemolytic transfusion reaction can also cause spherocytosis. In the neonatal period, consider haemolytic disease of the newborn, particularly that due to ABO incompatibility.

Hereditary elliptocytosis

The term hereditary elliptocytosis covers a heterogeneous group of inherited red cell membrane abnormalities characterized by elliptical red cells (see Fig. 2.14). Inheritance is usually autosomal dominant. Cases occur in many ethnic groups. Most cases are not anaemic and many do not have significant haemolysis.

The blood film shows elliptocytes and some ovalocytes. Polychromasia is usually absent. Cases with haemolytic anaemia have polychromasia and, in addition to elliptocytes and ovalo-cytes, often have other poikilocytes including some red cell fragments. In the great majority of cases the FBC is normal. Anaemic cases show a reduced Hb and increased RDW.

Further steps: The diagnosis of hereditary elliptocytosis can usually be made from the blood film. As haemolysis is unusual, further diagnostic tests are not usually necessary.

Glucose-6-phosphate dehydrogenase deficiency

Glucose-6-phosphate dehydrogenase (G6PD) is a red cell enzyme necessary to protect haemoglobin and other red cell proteins from endogenous or exogenous oxidant stress. Deficiency of G6PD leaves the individual susceptible to haemolysis during infection (endogenous oxidants generated by neutrophils) or on exposure to certain drugs, naphthalene in mothballs or fava beans (exogenous oxidants). Inheritance is sex-linked recessive. Cases occur in many ethnic groups but particularly in Africans, Afro-Caribbean, Afro-Americans, and in populations from the Middle East and around the Mediterranean. Most patients with a deficiency are haematologically normal between attacks of acute haemolysis.

During a haemolytic crisis the blood film (Fig. 4.7) shows irregularly contracted cells, keratocytes ('bite cells') and red cells with the haemoglobin retracted into half of the red cell mem-brane (hemighosts). The irregularly contracted cells often have protrusions that indicate the presence of Heinz bodies attached to the red cell membrane. Heinz bodies are red cell inclusions composed of denatured haemoglobin. They can be identified by a specific supravital stain. Heinz bodies and severely damaged red cells are removed by the spleen so that after a few days there are fewer irregularly contracted cells but polychromasia, indicative of a reticulocyte response, is then apparent.

Further steps: A test for Heinz bodies is not always necessary as it is often obvious from the very typical blood film that the patient has haemolysis induced by an oxidant. An assay for G6PD should be done. However, if the patient is already recover-

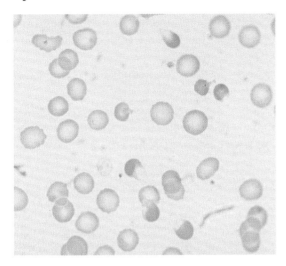

Fig. 4.7 Blood film during an acute haemolytic episode in glucose-6-phosphate dehydrogenase (G6PD) deficiency showing anaemia, irregularly contracted cells (some with protrusions) and a hemighost.

ing from the haemolysis and has a high reticulocyte count the result may be normal. This is particularly likely to occur with the type of G6PD deficiency that is found in those of African ethnic origin; they generally have normal levels of G6PD in reticulocytes although older cells are deficient; an episode of acute haemolysis can thus paradoxically lead to a rise in the G6PD concentration. Therefore, if the history and blood film suggest the possibility of G6PD deficiency but the assay is normal, repeat the test when the patient has recovered from the episode of haemolysis and the reticulocyte count has gone back to normal.

Autoimmune haemolytic anaemia

Autoimmune haemolytic anaemia is anaemia caused by autoantibodies, active at body temperature, directed at red antigens (warm autoantibodies). The condition is uncommon and can occur at any age.

The blood film (Fig. 4.8) shows spherocytosis and polychromatic macrocytes. The blood film in autoimmune haemolytic

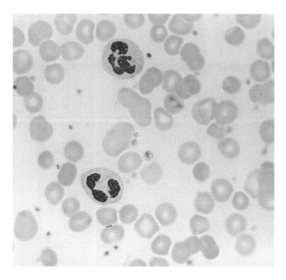

Fig. 4.8 Autoimmune haemolytic anaemia showing anaemia, spherocytosis and several polychromatic macrocytes.

anaemia cannot be reliably distinguished from that of hereditary spherocytosis, although anaemia and spherocytosis are often more severe than is usual in hereditary spherocytosis. Occasionally there are small red cell agglutinates or red cells that have been ingested by monocytes. The blood count shows the same abnormalities as are present in hereditary spherocytosis.

Further steps: Check the direct antiglobulin test (Coombs' test) to see if there is immunoglobulin or complement on the surface of the red cells. Test for antinuclear activity and for the presence of antibodies to double-stranded DNA, as an autoimmune haemolytic anaemia is often a feature of systemic lupus erythematosus.

Beta thalassaemia major

Beta thalassaemia major is a severe, transfusion-dependent anaemia resulting from homozygosity or compound heterozygosity for beta thalassaemia ($\beta^0\beta^0$ or $\beta^0\beta^+$ or $\beta^+\beta^+$). It occurs in all the ethnic groups with a significant incidence of beta thalassaemia trait. Clinical features are those of severe anaemia and, in addition, hepatomegaly, splenomegaly and overexpansion of marrow-containing bones.

The blood film shows striking anisocytosis, poikilocytosis, hypochromia and microcytosis. Poikilocytes include target cells. Red cells often contain Pappenheimer bodies and show basophilic stippling. In patients who have also been splenectomized, Pappenheimer bodies are very numerous and Howell–Jolly bodies are present. Sometimes there are precipitates with the same staining characteristics as haemoglobin; these are alpha chain precipitates, formed because of the lack of the beta globin chains that would normally combine with the alpha chains. NRBC are common. They show defective haemoglobinization and dysplastic features such as nuclear lobulation and fragmentation. There is marked reduction of the RBC, Hb, PCV/Hct, MCV and MCH. The MCHC is also reduced and the RDW is increased.

In patients who are being transfused (Fig. 4.9) there will be a mixture of normal transfused cells and the patient's cells showing the above abnormalities.

Further steps: In the absence of transfusion, beta thalassaemia major is incompatible with life so the diagnosis is usually made in infancy. The affected infants are found to become anaemic from around 6 months of life, as synthesis of fetal haemoglobin stops and synthesis of adequate amounts of haemoglobin A does not occur. The infant requires haemoglobin electrophoresis or high performance liquid chromatography (HPLC). This will show either no haemoglobin A or only small amounts with the only haemoglobin present in significant amounts being haemoglobin F. Both parents should be tested for beta thalassaemia trait and genetic counselling should be given. Beyond the neonatal period, the differential diagnosis is with beta thalassaemia intermedia. This is a genetically heterogeneous group of disorders that are more severe than beta thalassaemia trait but are compatible with life, even if not transfused.

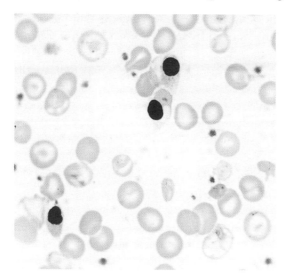

Fig. 4.9 Dimorphic blood film in a patient with thalassaemia major who was being transfused. The transfused red cells appear normal whereas the patient's red cells show hypochromia, anisocytosis, poikilocytosis and Pappenheimer bodies. One hypochromic cell (bottom right) contains an alpha chain precipitate. There are three NRBC, which show cytoplasmic defects consequent on the failure of haemoglobin synthesis.

Sickle cell anaemia

Sickle cell anaemia results from homozygosity for an abnormal beta globin gene, the β^s gene. As there is no normal beta gene there is no synthesis of normal beta globin and consequently no haemoglobin A can be produced. The haemoglobin is almost all haemoglobin S with a small amount of haemoglobin A_2 and a variable, sometimes increased, amount of haemoglobin F. Sickle cell anaemia is commonest in those of African ancestry but occurs also in other ethnic groups including Indians, Arabs and Greeks. The most prominent clinical feature is recurrent painful crises caused by tissue infarction.

The blood film in sickle cell anaemia (see Fig. 2.21) shows anaemia, sickle cells, boat-shaped cells and target cells. Once infancy is past, the changes of hyposplenism are also present, as a result of splenic infarction. Most striking is the presence of Howell–Jolly bodies but there are also some Pappenheimer bodies. NRBC are usually present and the WBC, neutrophil count, lymphocyte count and platelet count are often elevated. Polychromasia is usually present. The lack of polychromasia in sickle cell anaemia is a significant finding since it may indicate that red cell production has ceased and severe anaemia is developing, usually as a consequence of intercurrent parvovirus B19 infection.

The blood count usually shows an Hb of 7–9 g/dl. Some patients have a reduced MCV and MCH. The RDW is increased.

Further steps: Do haemoglobin electrophoresis or HPLC analysis to demonstrate the absence of haemoglobin A and the presence of mainly haemoglobin S with some haemoglobin A_2 and F. Check parents and confirm that both carry haemoglobin S. If the MCV and MCH are normal or near normal the diagnosis of sickle cell anaemia is confirmed but if the patient has microcytic red cells the diagnosis could also be compound heterozygosity for haemoglobin S and beta^0 thalassaemia. Family studies may permit the distinction but if this is not possible DNA analysis can be carried out. In an emergency, the diagnosis of sickle cell anaemia can be made fairly reliably by consideration of the Hb, red cell indices, blood film and sickle solubility test.

Sickle cell trait

Sickle cell trait is an asymptomatic condition consequent on heterozygosity for the β^s gene. Haemoglobin S and haemoglobin A are present in similar amounts although there is somewhat more haemoglobin A than haemoglobin S. The blood film may either be normal or show microcytosis or target cells. The FBC may be normal or show microcytosis. Since both the blood film and the blood count may be normal it is clear that the diagnosis of sickle cell trait cannot be based on either but requires specific tests for its detection.

Further steps: Haemoglobin electrophoresis or HPLC is required. The nature of a variant haemoglobin with characteristics suggestive of haemoglobin S on one of these tests must be confirmed by a sickle solubility test or by use of two independent methods, e.g. *both* haemoglobin electrophoresis *and* HPLC.

Sickle cell trait (haemoglobin S less than 50%) has to be distinguished from sickle cell/beta+ thalassaemia compound heterozygosity (haemoglobin S greater than 50%).

In an emergency, sickle cell trait can be provisionally diagnosed from the Hb, red cell indices, blood film and sickle solubility test. Sickle cell/haemoglobin C compound heterozygosity can also have a normal Hb and red cell indices but the blood film is much more abnormal than that of sickle cell trait (see below).

Sickle cell/haemoglobin C disease

Patients who are compound heterozygotes for haemoglobin S and haemoglobin C have these two haemoglobins in approximately equal amounts. Since they have no normal beta genes they cannot produce haemoglobin A. Sickle cell/haemoglobin C disease occurs in those with West African ancestry (since haemoglobin C originated in West Africa). Symptoms can be similar to those of sickle cell anaemia but are usually milder.

The blood film shows target cells, irregularly contracted cells and boat-shaped cells but classic sickle cells are much less frequent than in sickle cell anaemia. Many patients have a variable number of typical poikilocytes containing both haemoglobin S and haemoglobin C (SC poikilocytes) (see Fig. 2.22). There may be NRBC, polychromasia and features of hyposplenism but these are all less prominent than in sickle cell anaemia. Rare red cells may be found containing haemoglobin C crystals, recognized by their parallel edges. The FBC may show a normal Hb or a mild anaemia, the Hb being generally higher than 8 g/dl. Some patients have a reduced MCV and some have an elevated MCHC.

Further steps: Haemoglobin electrophoresis or HPLC, supplemented by a sickle solubility test, is required. Two independent tests are required to confirm the diagnosis.

Haemoglobin C disease

Haemoglobin C disease is consequent on homozygosity for an abnormal beta gene, β^C. There is no haemoglobin A. This condition occurs in people of West African ancestry. There is a chronic haemolytic anaemia, which may be asymptomatic or lead to gallstones.

The blood film (see Fig. 2.13) usually shows a mixture of target cells and irregularly contracted cells. Rare cells may contain haemoglobin C crystals. The FBC usually shows a mild to moderate anaemia. The MCV and MCH are often reduced and the MCHC is often increased.

Further steps: Haemoglobin electrophoresis or HPLC is required. Two independent tests are required to confirm the diagnosis. If there is microcytosis, an alternative diagnosis of haemoglobin C/beta^0 thalassaemia must be considered.

Abnormalities of white cells

Neutrophil leucocytosis (neutrophilia)

An increased neutrophil count is usually caused by increased bone marrow output. However, it can also be caused both by mobilization of the marginated granulocyte pool (neutrophils which have been adherent to the endothelium), e.g. following vigorous exercise or an epileptic fit, and by decreasing egress of neutrophils to the tissues, e.g. after administration of high doses of corticosteroids. Some important causes of neutrophil leucocytosis are shown in Table 4.4.

Bacterial infection

Most patients with bacterial infection have a neutrophil leucocytosis. The blood film may also show a left shift, toxic granulation, Döhle bodies and vacuolation (Fig. 4.10). There may be small numbers of atypical lymphocytes (e.g. plasmacytoid lymphocytes). There is lymphopenia and eosinopenia. If the bacterial infection becomes more chronic there may also be monocytosis, anaemia and increased rouleaux formation.

It is important not to misinterpret the physiological changes of pregnancy and the post-partum period as being due to infection. It should also be noted that all the changes characteristic of

Table 4.4 Some important causes of neutrophil leucocytosis.

Physiological and pharmacological
  Neonatal period, pregnancy and the post-partum period
  Mobilization of marginated granulocyte pool – exercise, epinephrine
    (adrenaline) injection, epileptic convulsions
  Administration of cytokines, e.g. granulocyte or granulocyte–
    macrophage colony-stimulating factors (G-CSF or GM-CSF)
  Administration of high-dose corticosteroids or lithium

Reactive
  Infection (particular bacterial infection)
  Tissue infarction (e.g. myocardial infarction)
  Other tissue damage (e.g. trauma, surgery, burns)
  Acute inflammation
  Acute haemorrhage or hypoxia

Neoplastic
  Leukaemia (particularly chronic myeloid leukaemia)
  Myeloproliferative disorders

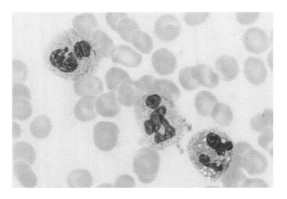

Fig. 4.10 Blood film in acute infection showing neutrophil leucocytosis, toxic granulation and vacuolation.

infection can be caused by the administration of granulocyte and granulocyte–macrophage colony-stimulating factors.

Further steps: Consider the clinical setting to exclude causes of neutrophilia other than bacterial infection. Look for other blood film features typical of bacterial infection.

Chronic myeloid leukaemia

Chronic myeloid leukaemia (also called chronic granulocytic leukaemia because the main cells produced are granulocytes) is a distinctive neoplastic condition, which, in the great majority of cases, is associated with a specific acquired cytogenetic abnormality in all myeloid cells. This is a translocation between chromosomes 9 and 22, known as t(9;22), leading to the formation of an abbreviated chromosome 22 known as the Philadelphia (Ph) chromosome.

Chronic myeloid leukaemia occurs at any age, mainly from late adolescence to old age. The disease is rare in children but occasional cases do occur. Clinically there is marked splenomegaly and a lesser degree of hepatomegaly.

The blood film is very characteristic (Fig. 4.11) and a correct diagnosis can usually be made from the blood count and film alone. There is a marked leucocytosis with the most frequent cells being myelocytes and mature neutrophils. There is a less marked increase in metamyelocytes, promyelocytes and blast cells. Basophils are increased in number in virtually all cases and eosinophils in about 80% of cases. Monocytes are increased,

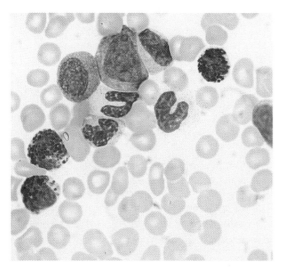

Fig. 4.11 Chronic myeloid (chronic granulocytic) leukaemia showing three basophils, an eosinophil myelocyte and mature and immature cells of neutrophil lineage.

but not in proportion to cells of the granulocyte lineages. There is usually a mild to moderate normocytic, normochromic anaemia. The platelet count is most often normal or increased but is occasionally reduced. The white cells do not usually show any dysplastic features, nor are there any reactive or 'toxic' features such as toxic granulation, Döhle bodies or neutrophil vacuolation.

Further steps: A very accurate diagnosis is required because there is now very specific treatment for this type of leukaemia. All patients in whom the diagnosis is suspected require cytogenetic analysis of bone marrow cells to detect the t(9;22) translocation. If it is not detected but the suspicion of the diagnosis is strong, molecular genetic analysis is also needed to see if the fusion gene that usually results from a t(9;22) translocation (*BCR–ABL* fusion) is present despite the absence of the translocation.

Chronic myeloid leukaemia is not usually confused with reactive neutrophilia, e.g. as a response to infection, because an increase in the eosinophil and basophil counts does not generally occur in infection, the number of granulocyte precursors in the blood is generally less and reactive changes such as toxic granulation, are often present.

Lymphocytosis and morphologically abnormal lymphoid cells

Lymphocytosis can be caused by increased mobilization of lymphocytes from tissues into the blood stream or by increased production of lymphocytes, either in response to an antigenic stimulus or as a neoplastic condition. Transient lymphocytosis, due to redistribution of lymphocytes, occurs as an acute response to severe physical stress. When there is lymphocytosis as a response to an infection there are often also morphological changes in lymphocytes; these are most striking in infectious mononucleosis, in which atypical lymphocytes (see Fig. 3.9) are numerous. More subtle reactive changes in lymphocytes are common in other infections, particular infections in children or viral infections at any age. Lymphoid cells are also morphologically abnor-

Table 4.5 Some important causes of lymphocytosis.

Physiological and caused by kinetic alterations
Exercise
Epinephrine (adrenaline) administration
As an early acute reaction to physical stress (e.g. following trauma,
sickle cell crisis, myocardial infarction, cardiac arrest)

Reactive
Infections [particularly viral and rickettsial infections,
whooping-cough (pertussis), bacterial infections in infants and
young children]

Neoplastic
Chronic lymphocytic leukaemia
Other lymphoid leukaemias
Lymphomas in leukaemic phases

mal in lymphoid neoplasms. Some of the important causes of
lymphocytosis are shown in Table 4.5.

Further steps: Assess the clinical history and physical findings.
Has there been sudden severe physical stress? Are there signs or
symptoms of infection, such as fever or sore throat? Is there
enlargement of lymph nodes, liver or spleen, suggestive of a
lymphoproliferative disorder? The blood count needs to be repeated to exclude transient lymphocytosis. Persistent lymphocytosis is usually an indication for immunophenotyping the cells
to facilitate diagnosis of a lymphoproliferative disorder.

Chronic lymphocytic leukaemia

Chronic lymphocytic leukaemia is a disease of the middle-aged
and elderly. In the early stages of the disease there may be no
abnormal physical findings. Later there is lymphadenopathy,
hepatomegaly and splenomegaly.

The blood film in chronic lymphocytic leukaemia (Fig. 4.12) is
characterized by an increase of small, mature lymphocytes
(which are of B lineage). In the early stages the lymphocyte count
is only moderately elevated but later the count may be very high.

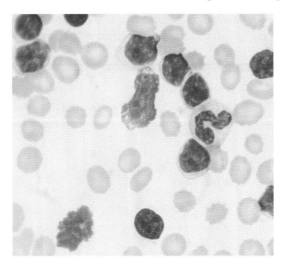

Fig. 4.12 Chronic lymphocytic leukaemia, showing lymphocytosis with an increase of mature small lymphocytes. There are two smear cells.

The cells are more uniform in appearance than normal small lymphocytes. Both the cell and the nucleus have a smooth regular outline. The nucleocytoplasmic ratio is high. The nuclear chromatin is usually moderately condensed and nucleoli are not usually apparent. Often nuclear chromatin is coarsely clumped, giving a mosaic or paving-stone pattern. The cytoplasm is agranular but occasionally contains crystals or globular inclusions. Smear cells, formed when the cell is disrupted during the spreading of the film, are characteristic but not pathognomonic. In some patients there is anaemia or thrombocytopenia. Anaemia can be caused by complicating autoimmune haemolytic anaemia and in these cases spherocytes are apparent.

Further steps: If the lymphocytosis is persistent, immunophenotyping is usually indicated to confirm the diagnosis, even if the patient does not have lymphadenopathy or hepatosplenomegaly. However, elderly patients with early disease need to be reassured as disease progression is often slow and they may not need treatment for many years, if at all. Nevertheless, confirming the diagnosis means that the patient's general practitioner is alert to the possibility of common complications, such as herpes zoster, that may need treatment. A bone marrow aspirate and trephine biopsy does not yield much information in the early stages of the disease, but these investigations are indicated if there is a possibility that the patient will soon need treatment. If there are spherocytes, a direct antiglobulin test is indicated to confirm the presence of complicating autoimmune haemolytic anaemia.

Prolymphocytic leukaemia

Prolymphocytic leukaemia is a disease of the middle-aged and elderly. Clinically there is marked splenomegaly and minor lymphadenopathy.

The WBC is usually markedly elevated and there is an increase of lymphoid cells, which are morphologically very abnormal (Fig. 4.13). They are larger than normal lymphocytes with a large and prominent nucleolus. The chromatin shows irregular condensation.

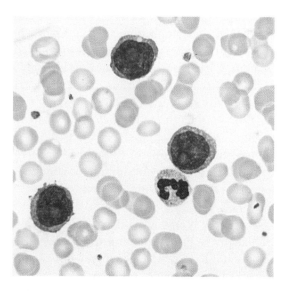

Fig. 4.13 Prolymphocytic leukaemia (B-lineage) showing three prolymphocytes. These cells are larger than the cells of chronic lymphocytic leukaemia and have large, prominent nucleoli.

Further steps: Immunophenotyping is indicated to confirm that there is a clonal B-cell population.

Follicular lymphoma

Lymphomas are lymphoid neoplasms that predominantly affect lymph nodes and other lymphoid tissues. However, lymphomas may infiltrate the bone marrow and there may be an overspill of lymphoma cells into the blood. Follicular lymphoma is a disease of adult life. It is characterized clinically by lymphadenopathy, splenomegaly or both, and pathologically by a nodular or follicular growth pattern of neoplastic cells in lymph nodes. A significant minority of patients have circulating lymphoma cells.

Follicular lymphoma cells are usually smaller than the cells of chronic lymphocytic leukaemia and more pleomorphic. They have very scanty cytoplasm. The nucleus shows a more even chromatin distribution. Some cells have distinctive notches or deep clefts (Fig. 4.14). Patients may have only small numbers of circulating lymphoma cells or the abnormal cells may be sufficiently numerous to cause a lymphocytosis. In those cases with lymphocytosis it is important to note the distinctive cellular features to avoid confusion with chronic lymphocytic leukaemia.

Further steps: Immunophenotyping is indicated to confirm that there is a clonal B-cell population. Lymph node biopsy may

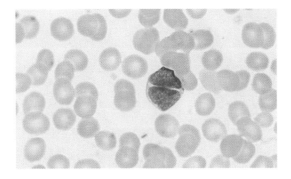

Fig. 4.14 Cleft lymphocyte in follicular lymphoma.

be needed to confirm the diagnosis. However, specific cytogenetic and molecular genetic abnormalities are found in follicular lymphoma and these analyses, together with immunophenotyping, can confirm the diagnosis and obviate the need for a general anaesthetic for a lymph node biopsy.

Hairy cell leukaemia

Hairy cell leukaemia is a B-lineage lymphoid neoplasm with distinctive neoplastic cells. It is a disease of adult life characterized clinically by splenomegaly without lymphadenopathy.

Hairy cells (Fig. 4.15) are larger than normal lymphocytes. The nucleus is often round but is sometimes lobulated or shaped like a peanut shell or a dumbbell. There is moderately plentiful, weakly basophilic cytoplasm with irregular 'hairy' margins. Hairy cells are usually present only in small numbers so a careful search may be necessary to find and identify them. Pancytopenia is usual with neutropenia being common and monocytopenia being particularly severe.

Further steps: Immunophenotyping is indicated to confirm that there is a clonal B-cell population with a distinctive immunophenotype. Cytochemistry, to demonstrate tartrate-resistant acid phosphatase activity, can also confirm the diagnosis when considered in conjunction with the cytological features. A trephine biopsy is also diagnostically useful, showing characteristically widely spaced cells.

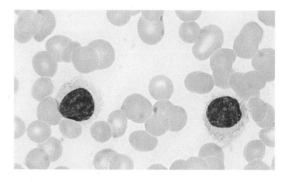

Fig. 4.15 Two hairy cells in hairy cell leukaemia.

Multiple myeloma

Multiple myeloma is a plasma cell neoplasm in which the malignant cells usually secrete an abnormal immunoglobulin known as a paraprotein. The main site of disease is the bone marrow and bones. Multiple myeloma is predominantly a disease of the middle-aged and elderly. Common clinical features are anaemia, bone pain, pathological fractures, hypercalcaemia and renal failure.

In the majority of patients the blood film shows increased rouleaux formation and increased background staining between the cells. Both are caused by the increased concentration of immunoglobulin in the blood. There is a normocytic, normochromic anaemia. Occasionally there are circulating myeloma cells (see Fig. 2.4), which resemble normal plasma cells to a greater or lesser extent, i.e. they may have plentiful basophilic cytoplasm, an eccentric nucleus and a paler-staining zone in the cytoplasm adjacent to the nucleus representing the Golgi zone.

Detecting the features of multiple myeloma in patients with a normocytic normochromic anaemia can be very important in patient management, as this is often the first clue to the nature of the patient's illness.

Further steps: The suspicion of multiple myeloma requires: a bone marrow aspirate and trephine biopsy, investigations for a serum paraprotein and for urinary monoclonal immunoglobulin light chains (Bence–Jones protein), measurement of the concentration of normal serum immunoglobulin and radiographs of relevant bones, including the skull (a 'skeletal survey'). Occasionally magnetic resonance imaging (MRI), to image the bone marrow, may be necessary.

The acute leukaemias and related conditions

The acute leukaemias are characterized by proliferation of immature cells, either lymphoid or myeloid, with a failure of differentiation to mature end cells. Because the immature cells are proliferating in the bone marrow they replace normal haemopoietic cells and cause anaemia and various cytopenias. Proliferation of leukaemic cells in other organs causes some degree of hepatomegaly and splenomegaly and, particularly in the case of acute lymphoblastic leukaemia, lymphadenopathy.

Acute lymphoblastic leukaemia

Acute lymphoblastic leukaemia is predominantly a disease of children. It is caused by proliferation, in the bone marrow and lymphoid tissues, of lymphoblasts of either B or T lineage. Overspill into the blood occurs in the majority of cases. Patients are often anaemic or thrombocytopenic. Acute lymphoblastic leukaemia has been divided into three morphological subtypes L1, L2 and L3 by an international cooperative group, the French–American–British (FAB) group. Most childhood cases have L1 morphology (Fig. 4.16). The blasts are fairly uniform in appearance but vary in size from that of a normal lymphocyte to about twice this size. They have a high nucleocytoplasmic ratio, a delicate diffuse chromatin pattern and sometimes small nucleoli.

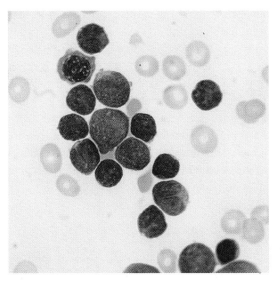

Fig. 4.16 Acute lymphoblastic leukaemia of L1 subtype. There is one NRBC; all the other cells are lymphoblasts.

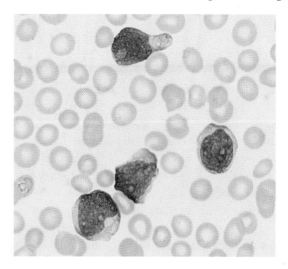

Fig. 4.17 Acute lymphoblastic leukaemia of L2 subtype.

The smaller blasts can show some chromatin condensation. Some childhood cases and a larger proportion of adult cases have L2 morphology (Fig. 4.17). The blasts are larger than those of L1, have more plentiful cytoplasm and are more pleomorphic. Both cells and nuclei may be irregular in shape and nucleoli are sometimes prominent. A small minority of cases have L3 morphology (Fig. 4.18). Cells are fairly regular in shape. They have moderately to strongly basophilic cytoplasm and prominent cytoplasmic

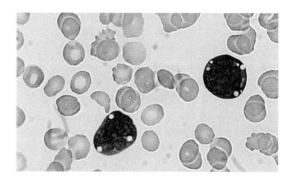

Fig. 4.18 Acute lymphoblastic leukaemia of L3 subtype (can also be regarded as the leukaemic equivalent of Burkitt's lymphoma).

vacuolation in at least a proportion of cells. Whether blast cells have L1 or L2 features is of little clinical significance. L1 acute lymphoblastic leukaemia can usually be readily diagnosed from the cytological features alone, whereas L2 acute lymphoblastic leukaemia is more likely to be confused with acute myeloid leukaemia and special tests to make the distinction are important. Otherwise, this categorization can be ignored. The L3 subtype, however, has a very specific clinical significance. Cytological features are the same as in the leukaemic phase of Burkitt's lymphoma. L3 morphology correlates with a mature B cell immunophenotype and requires specific management. In fact, the most recent classification of acute leukaemia, that proposed by the World Health Organization expert group, classifies this condition as a leukaemic phase of non-Hodgkin's lymphoma rather than as acute leukaemia. This is appropriate since, although the disease is clinically very aggressive, the immunophenotype is that of a mature B cell rather than that of a B-cell precursor.

Further steps: When facilities are available, immunophenotyping is always indicated in suspected acute lymphoblastic leukaemia. This is for two reasons; (i) to distinguish the blast cells of T- or B-lineage acute lymphoblastic leukaemia from the blast cells of some acute myeloid leukaemias with very primitive myeloblasts; and (ii) to distinguish non-Hodgkin's lymphoma (mature B or T cells) from acute lymphoblastic leukaemia/lymphoblastic lymphoma (B- or T-cell precursors).

These are very important distinctions to make since the treatment is very different. In addition, if facilities are available, cytogenetic and molecular analysis are indicated in all cases of acute lymphoblastic leukaemia. This is because all cases are not the same. There are many sub-types that require individual management. Cytochemistry is irrelevant in acute lymphoblastic leukaemia unless immunophenotyping is unavailable.

Acute myeloid leukaemia

Acute myeloid leukaemia occurs at all ages from the neonatal period to old age. However, the incidence increases steadily

Table 4.6 Simplified FAB classification of acute myeloid leukaemia.

M0	Acute myeloblastic leukaemia with minimal evidence of myeloid differentiation
M1	Acute myeloid leukaemia with little maturation beyond the myeloblast stage
M2	Acute myeloid leukaemia with maturation
M3	Acute hypergranular promyelocytic leukaemia (M3) and its microgranular or hypogranular variant (M3 variant)
M4	Acute myelomonocytic leukaemia
M5	Acute monoblastic (M5a) and monocytic (M5b) leukaemia
M6	Acute erythroleukaemia
M7	Acute megakaryoblastic leukaemia

through adult life and old age. Acute myeloid leukaemia has been divided by the FAB group into eight morphological subtypes, which are summarized, in a simplified form, in Table 4.6. Diagnosis and classification of acute myeloid leukaemia require examination of a bone marrow aspirate but, since blast cells are usually present in the blood, a provisional diagnosis can often be made from examination of the blood film. It is necessary to recognize myeloblasts, monoblasts and normal and abnormal promyelocytes in order to recognize and classify acute myeloid leukaemia. In M0 and M1 acute myeloid leukaemia the predominant cell is a myeloblast. It is a large cell with a high nucleocytoplasmic ratio. One or more nucleoli may be detected in the nucleus. In M1 acute myeloid leukaemia the cytoplasm may contain scanty granules or Auer rods (Fig. 4.19). In M2 acute myeloid leukaemia promyelocytes are also present (Fig. 4.20). They have more numerous granules than myeloblasts and may have an eccentric nucleus and a Golgi zone. In M4 acute myeloid leukaemia both myeloblasts and monoblasts are present (Fig. 4.21). Monoblasts are larger than myeloblasts with voluminous cytoplasm. Cytoplasmic basophilia varies from weak to moderately strong. The cytoplasm is sometimes vacuolated. The monoblast may be a round cell with a round nucleus or irregular in shape with a lobulated nucleus. There is often a large nucleolus. In M5 acute myeloid leukaemia the dominant cell may be a monoblast (M5a) or there may also be promonocytes and mature monocytes (M5b). Promonocytes are larger than monocytes and

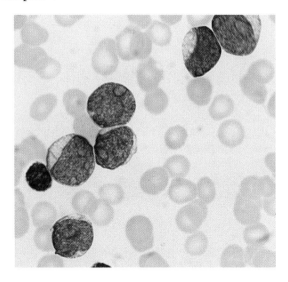

Fig. 4.19 Acute myeloid leukaemia of M1 subtype showing six myeloblasts and a lymphocyte. The blast cell adjacent to the lymphocyte contains an Auer rod.

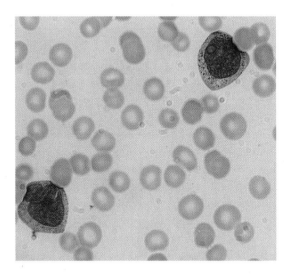

Fig. 4.20 Acute myeloid leukaemia of M2 subtype showing two promyelocytes.

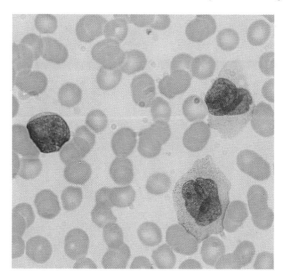

Fig. 4.21 Acute myeloid leukaemia of M4 subtype showing a myeloblast (left) and two monoblasts (right).

have more basophilic and heavily granulated cytoplasm. M3 acute myeloid leukaemia (Fig. 4.22) is cytologically very distinctive. The promyelocyte cytoplasm is packed with large, brightly staining azurophilic granules. There may be giant granules or bundles of Auer rods. M3 variant acute myeloid leukaemia is more difficult to diagnose on cytological features, particularly from the peripheral blood film. By light microscopy most of the promyelocytes have no apparent granules but a minority have fine dust-like granules, a pink blush to the cytoplasm or bundles of Auer rods. Many of the promyelocytes have a distinctive bilobed nucleus (Fig. 4.23).

Most cases of acute myeloid leukaemia have a normocytic, normochromic anaemia and thrombocytopenia. A small minority of cases have an increased platelet count. Neutropenia is also characteristic but some cases of M2 acute myeloid leukaemia have neutrophilia. A very small minority of cases have eosinophilia or basophilia. M0 and M7 acute myeloid leukaemia cannot be distinguished from acute lymphoblastic leukaemia by microscopy alone. Diagnosis of M6 acute myeloid leukaemia always requires bone marrow examination.

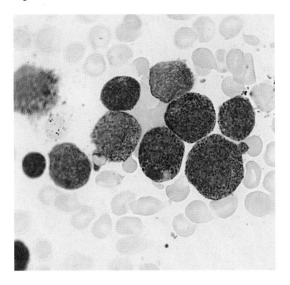

Fig. 4.22 Acute myeloid leukaemia of M3 subtype showing hypergranular promyelocytes, one of which contains a giant granule.

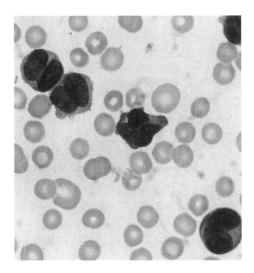

Fig. 4.23 Acute myeloid leukaemia of M3 variant subtype showing the characteristic bilobed hypogranular promyelocytes.

Further steps: If acute myeloid leukaemia is suspected, cytochemistry is needed to confirm the myeloid nature of the abnormal cells (if this is not already obvious). A bone marrow aspirate and cytogenetic analysis are also needed, since the cytogenetic sub-type is increasingly used in planning optimal treatment for each individual patient. Immunophenotyping is sometimes needed, to confirm a diagnosis of acute myeloid rather than acute lymphoblastic leukaemia. This is necessarily so in the FAB category of M0 acute myeloid leukaemia, in which the blast cells are very primitive and do not express myeloperoxidase, nonspecific esterase or other myeloid enzymes. They do, however, express antigens that are characteristic of myeloid cells. Immunophenotyping may also be necessary in cases of acute myeloid leukaemia in which the leukaemic blast cells are megakaryoblasts (M7 acute myeloid leukaemia).

If M3 or M3 variant acute myeloid leukaemia is suspected, it is vital to confirm the diagnosis rapidly. This is because this condition is often complicated by disseminated intravascular coagulation and there is a need for urgent correction of the coagulation abnormality and specific anti-leukaemic treatment. An accurate as well as a speedy diagnosis of this subtype of acute leukaemia is particularly important since the specific treatment indicated differs from that in other types of acute myeloid leukaemia.

The myelodysplastic syndromes

The myelodysplastic syndromes are related to acute myeloid leukaemia. Both are neoplasms of myeloid cells with continued proliferation of myeloid precursors but defective production of mature end cells. In the myelodysplastic syndromes the dissociation between proliferation and maturation is not as severe as in acute myeloid leukaemia so that some end cells are produced. However, haemopoiesis is ineffective, leading to the paradox of frequent pancytopenia (anaemia, leucopenia and thrombocytopenia) despite a cellular bone marrow. Blast cells may be increased and acute myeloid leukaemia may supervene in patients with one of the myelodysplastic syndromes. This group of closely related conditions occurs mainly in the elderly.

The blood film shows various cytopenias, most often anaemia, neutropenia and thrombocytopenia. Blood cells are often morphologically abnormal. Red cells may be macrocytic or, in those with defective incorporation of iron into haemoglobin, there may be a minor population of hypochromic microcytes and Pappenheimer bodies (see Fig. 2.23). Neutrophils may be hypogranular (see Fig. 1.13) or show the acquired Pelger–Huët anomaly. Platelets may show abnormal variation in size or be hypogranular or agranular. Blasts may be present and occasionally they contain Auer rods. Monocytes may be increased. The neutrophil count may be increased but neutropenia is much more common. The platelet count is increased in a minority of patients but is more often decreased.

Further steps: Bone marrow aspiration is required, to assess the number of blast cells and exclude a diagnosis of acute myeloid leukaemia. This should be supplemented by cytogenetic analysis, which sometimes confirms an otherwise uncertain diagnosis and in other instances gives information of prognostic importance. Cytochemical stains are indicated on the bone marrow aspirate, to detect any ring sideroblasts (Perls' stain) or Auer rods (Sudan Black B or myeloperoxidase stain) that might be present. Since non-neoplastic conditions can also cause dysplastic changes in haemopoietic cells, it is sometimes necessary to exclude other conditions before making a presumptive diagnosis of myelodysplastic syndrome. Such conditions include alcohol and drug toxicity, vitamin B_{12} or folic acid deficiency, heavy metal exposure and human immunodeficiency virus (HIV) infection.

Idiopathic myelofibrosis

Idiopathic myelofibrosis is a myeloproliferative disorder with onset usually in middle or old age. The fibrosis that affects the bone marrow is a reactive change that results from the proliferation of a clone of neoplastic haemopoietic cells. It is therefore no longer 'idiopathic' but the name remains convenient, to distinguish this condition from secondary myelofibrosis. The blood film is important in suggesting the diagnosis. There is a normocytic, normochromic anaemia with marked anisocytosis and poikilocytosis. Teardrop poikilocytes are present. The blood film is leucoerythroblastic, i.e. NRBC and granulocyte precursors are present. In the early stages of the disease there may be neutrophilia or thrombocytosis but usually there is pancytopenia. Platelets may show increased variation in size and granularity with some poorly granulated platelets and some giant forms. Occasionally circulating megakaryocytes or megakaryocyte bare nuclei are present.

Further steps: The blood film in idiopathic myelofibrosis cannot be distinguished from that in myelofibrosis secondary to other myeloproliferative disorders (e.g. polycythaemia vera or essential thrombocythaemia). Knowledge of the previous history is essential to make the distinction. The differential diagnosis also includes secondary myelofibrosis due to bone marrow infiltration in metastatic carcinoma. Assessment of clinical features is very important in making this distinction since splenomegaly is almost invariable in idiopathic myelofibrosis but is rare in metastatic carcinoma. A leucoerythroblastic blood film can also result from shock or acute hypoxia or reflect recovery from bone marrow suppression or recovery from haematinic deficiency (deficiency of iron, vitamin B_{12} or folic acid).

CHAPTER 5

Self-assessment

This self-assessment chapter contains questions of varying levels of difficulty. Most can be answered fully using the information in this book. However, the clinical questions, which are designed mainly for candidates preparing for higher examinations (e.g. of the Royal College of Pathologists and the Royal College of Physicians in the UK), are more difficult and most require extra knowledge. Nevertheless, since answers to the questions are given and discussed, all readers should benefit from thinking about all the questions.

Exercise 1 (for all readers)

Go through the book, covering the legends and identifying the features in the illustrations. Uncover the legends and check if you are right.

Exercise 2 (for medical students, trainee laboratory scientists and trainee haematologists)

Using blood films and a microscope identify the major morphological features discussed in this book and check your identification of cell types or morphological abnormalities with an experienced laboratory worker.

Exercise 3 (for trainee laboratory scientists and trainee haematologists)

Select some patient blood films, examine the blood films

microscopically, assess the blood counts and decide what you would write on a report form to be sent back to clinical staff. Compare what you have written with the reports written by senior laboratory staff and discuss any discrepancy with them.

Exercise 4 – multiple choice questions (for all readers)

Answer the following true or false questions and then compare your answers with those on pages 102–104. (It is suggested that you photostat the relevant pages rather than writing in the book. Fill in the circle for each true answer.) The number of correct answers may be zero to five.

Q1 Microcytosis is characteristic of:

1 Beta thalassaemia trait . . . . O
2 Iron deficiency anaemia . . . . O
3 Depletion of body iron stores without anaemia . . . . O
4 Hereditary elliptocytosis . . . . O
5 Megaloblastic anaemia . . . . O

Q2 A 23-year-old Cypriot woman has a blood count for premarital counselling. The results are as follows: RBC $5.5 \times 10^{12}/l$, Hb 13.0 g/dl, PCV 0.38, MCV 70 fl, MCH 23.6 pg, MCHC 34.2 g/dl, RDW 14. Which of the following possibilities is *most* likely:

1 The patient is haematologically normal . . . . O
2 Body iron stores are depleted . . . . O
3 She has beta thalassaemia trait . . . . O
4 She has congenital sideroblastic anaemia . . . . O
5 She has sickle cell trait . . . . O

Q3 Macrocytosis may be a feature of:

1 Chronic haemolytic anaemia . . . . O
2 Excess alcohol intake . . . . O
3 Hyperthyroidism . . . . O

4 Myelodysplastic syndromes .... ○
5 Sickle cell trait .... ○

Q4 Neutrophil leucocytosis is likely to occur in:

1 Myocardial infarction .... ○
2 Whooping-cough (pertussis) .... ○
3 Sickle cell crisis .... ○
4 Hypersplenism .... ○
5 Chronic granulocytic leukaemia .... ○

Q5 The following are likely 1 day after major surgery:

1 Neutrophil leucocytosis .... ○
2 Left shift .... ○
3 Lymphocytopenia .... ○
4 Eosinopenia .... ○
5 Toxic granulation .... ○

Q6 The following may be a feature of sickle cell trait:

1 Target cells .... ○
2 Sickle cells .... ○
3 Neutrophil leucocytosis .... ○
4 Macrocytosis .... ○
5 Polychromasia .... ○

Q7 Indicate whether the following statements about Döhle bodies are true or false:

1 They are a reliable indication of infection .... ○
2 They are composed of denatured haemoglobin .... ○
3 They are composed of DNA .... ○
4 They may occur in healthy pregnant women .... ○
5 They are likely to be associated with left shift and toxic
   granulation .... ○

Q8 The following groups are likely to have higher neutrophil counts than healthy adult Caucasian males:

1 Healthy Afro-Caribbean males . . . . ○
2 Pregnant women . . . . ○
3 Neonates . . . . ○
4 Patients who have just suffered an epileptic convulsion . . . ○
5 Patients being administered high doses of corticosteroids . . ○

Q9 The following can occur as a result of splenectomy:

1 Neutropenia . . . . ○
2 Thrombocytopenia . . . . ○
3 Howell–Jolly bodies . . . . ○
4 Target cells . . . . ○
5 Acanthocytes . . . . ○

Q10 The following are usually associated with spherocytes in the blood film:

1 Severe iron deficiency anaemia . . . . ○
2 Combined deficiency of vitamin B_{12} and folic acid . . . . ○
3 Severe burns . . . . ○
4 Autoimmune haemolytic anaemia . . . . ○
5 Polycythaemia rubra vera . . . . ○

Q11 The following may have target cells as a blood film feature:

1 Obstructive jaundice . . . . ○
2 Sickle cell trait . . . . ○
3 Sickle cell disease . . . . ○
4 Splenic atrophy . . . . ○
5 Haemoglobin C disease . . . . ○

Q12 The following may cause polycythaemia:

1 Living below sea level . . . . ○
2 Low-oxygen-affinity haemoglobin . . . . ○

3 Polycystic kidneys . . . . ○
4 Sleep apnoea . . . . ○
5 Morbid obesity . . . . ○

Answers to multiple choice questions

Q1 TTFFF

Discussion: Beta thalassaemia trait and iron deficiency anaemia are both characterized by microcytosis. Depletion of iron stores without anaemia does not cause microcytosis. In hereditary elliptocytosis the red cell indices are normal. Megaloblastic anaemia is characterized by macrocytosis, not microcytosis.

Q2 FFTFF

Discussion: The patient is not haematologically normal, as can be seen by comparing her red cell indices with the normal range for healthy adult women. Depletion of body iron stores does not cause microcytosis in advance of anaemia. Congenital sideroblastic anaemia is very unlikely since the patient is not anaemic and this rare condition occurs mainly in men. Sickle cell trait would be possible but it is unlikely in a Cypriot woman and the MCV is often normal. The red cell indices are typical of beta thalassaemia trait, which is common in Cyprus.

Q3 TTFTF

Discussion: Macrocytosis is characteristic of chronic haemolytic anaemia and alcohol excess. It is often present in the myelodysplastic syndromes. Macrocytosis is a feature of hypothyroidism, not hyperthyroidism. Sickle cell trait may be associated with microcytosis but macrocytosis is not a feature.

Q4 TFTFT

Discussion: Neutrophil leucocytosis is likely in myocardial infarction and sickle cell crisis, as a response to tissue infarction. It is unlikely in whooping-cough, in which the usual haematological abnormality is lymphocytosis. Hypersplenism is characterized by neutropenia rather than neutrophilia. Neutrophilia is invariable in chronic granulocytic leukaemia.

Q5 TTTTT

Discussion: All these abnormalities are part of the usual response to major surgery.

Q6 TFFFF

Discussion: The blood film in sickle cell trait is often normal. The only abnormalities which are at all likely are target cells and microcytosis. Sickle cells are not seen.

Q7 FFFTT

Discussion: Döhle bodies are cytoplasmic inclusions in neutrophils composed of ribosomes. They are not denatured haemoglobin (Heinz bodies) or DNA (Howell–Jolly bodies). They occur in infection, in inflammation, following cytokine administration and in pregnancy and so are not a reliable indication of infection. They are often associated with other reactive changes in neutrophils such as left shift and toxic granulation.

Q8 FTTTT

Discussion: Healthy Afro-Caribbean tend to have lower neutrophil counts than Caucasians, rather than higher. Pregnant women and neonates have a higher normal range than adult males. Epileptic convulsions mobilize the marginated granulocyte pool and thus raise the neutrophil count. Corticosteroids alter granulocyte kinetics and raise the neutrophil count.

Q9 FFTTT

Discussion: Splenectomy is likely to be associated with increased neutrophil and platelet counts rather than reduced counts. The other abnormalities are expected in hyposplenism.

Q10 FFTTF

Discussion: Severe thermal burns cause direct damage to the red cell membrane and lead to spherocyte formation. Warm red cell autoantibodies attach to the red cell membrane, leading to removal of part of the membrane in the spleen and consequent spherocyte formation. The other conditions listed do not cause spherocytosis.

Q11 TTTTT

Discussion: Target cells are sometimes present in sickle cell trait and are usually present in all the other conditions listed.

Q12 FFTTT

Discussion: Living at a *high* altitude and a *high*-affinity haemoglobin would be likely to cause polycythaemia. Renal cysts and tumour can lead to increased erythropoietin secretion and polycythaemia. Sleep apnoea and morbid obesity can both cause hypoxia and thus stimulate erythropoietin secretion and cause polycythaemia.

Exercise 5 – clinical cases (for all readers)

Q1 A 28-year-old Caucasian man presented with weight loss, sweating, fatigue and abdominal discomfort. He was found to be pale and his spleen was enlarged 15 cm below the left costal margin. WBC was 100 × 10⁹/l, Hb 10.0 g/dl and platelet count 600 × 10⁹/l. His blood film is illustrated in Fig. 5.1.

1 List the abnormalities shown.
2 What is the most likely diagnosis?
3 What is the single test most likely to be useful in diagnosis?
4 What other tests could be useful in diagnosis?

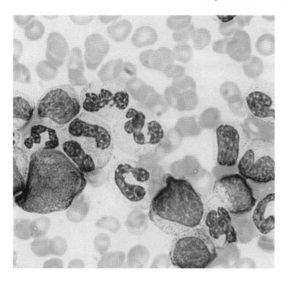

Fig. 5.1 Peripheral blood film (Exercise 5, Q1).

Q2 A 23-year-old woman had suffered for many years from recurrent pains in her limbs and abdomen. Her mother was Italian and was known to suffer from beta thalassaemia trait. Her father was Afro-Caribbean. Her Hb was 10 g/dl and MCV 70 fl. Her blood film is illustrated in Fig. 5.2.

1 List all the abnormalities shown.
2 What is the most likely diagnosis?
3 What tests would be most useful in diagnosis and what would you expect to find?
4 What abnormality if any would you expect to find in the patient's father?

Q3 A 40-year-old northern European Caucasian woman with dermatitis herpetiformis was being treated by her dermatologist with dapsone. She was noted to be pale and a blood count was therefore performed. This showed an Hb of 9.5 g/dl and an MCV of 110 fl. Her blood film is illustrated in Fig. 5.3.

1 List all the abnormalities present.
2 What is the most likely diagnosis?

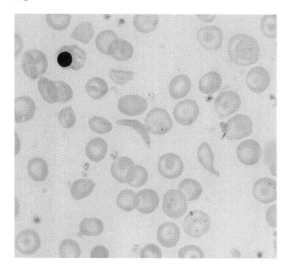

Fig. 5.2 Peripheral blood film (Exercise 5, Q2).

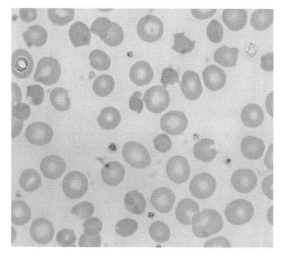

Fig. 5.3 Peripheral blood film (Exercise 5, Q3).

3 List the three tests which would be most useful in confirming the diagnosis, assessing the severity of the conditions and managing the patient.

Q4 An 18-year-old Caucasian university student presented to his general practitioner with fever, marked cervical lymphadenopathy and malaise. He was found to have large inflamed tonsils and slight jaundice. His WBC was $15 \times 10^9/l$ and his platelet count $60 \times 10^9/l$. His blood film showed numerous atypical lymphocytes.

1 What is the most likely diagnosis?
2 What is the cause of this condition?
3 What test is usually done to confirm the diagnosis?

Q5 A 60-year-old Afro-Caribbean woman was referred to medical outpatients because of lethargy, fatigue and chronic backache. The only abnormality found on physical examination was pallor. Results of her FBC were: WBC $5.0 \times 10^9/l$, Hb 9.5 g/dl, MCV 95 fl, platelet count $120 \times 10^9/l$. Biochemical screening showed: total protein 84 g/l (normal range 60–80 g/l), albumin 33 g/l (normal range 35–51 g/l), serum calcium 2.6 mmol/l (normal range 2.15–2.55 mmol/l), creatinine 140 μmol/l (normal range 60–125 μmol/l). Her blood film is illustrated in Fig. 2.4 (see page 31).

1 What abnormalities are shown in the blood film?
2 What is the most likely diagnosis?
3 List the two tests most likely to confirm the diagnosis.
4 List the three abnormalities most likely to have contributed to the elevated serum creatinine.

Q6 A 5-year-old Caucasian boy presented with a history of a diarrhoeal illness followed by vomiting and mild jaundice. He was found to be anaemic and to have a greatly elevated serum creatinine. His blood film is illustrated in Fig. 5.4.

1 What abnormalities are shown in the blood film?
2 What is the general name for this type of anaemia?
3 What is the most likely diagnosis?

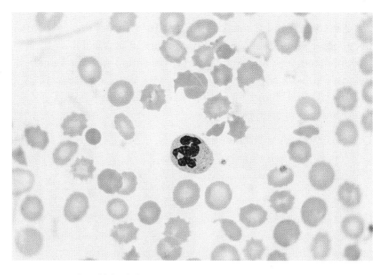

Fig. 5.4 Peripheral blood film (Exercise 5, Q6).

Q7 A 70-year-old Caucasian man presented to his general practitioner with a history of gradual onset of tiredness and bruising. His FBC was: WBC 4 × 10⁹/l, neutrophil count 0.8 × 10⁹/l, Hb 8.5 g/dl and platelet count 50 × 10⁹/l. His blood film is illustrated in Fig. 1.13 (see page 14).

1 List all the abnormalities shown in the blood film.
2 What is the most likely diagnosis?
3 What test is essential for confirmation of the diagnosis?
4 What supplementary test would give useful information?

Q8 A 30-year-old Caucasian woman presented to a casualty department with recent onset of nose bleeding. She was found to have multiple bruises and a blood count and coagulation screen were therefore performed. Results of the FBC were: WBC 8 × 10⁹/l, Hb 10.5 g/dl, platelet count 50 × 10⁹/l. The prothrombin time, activated thromboplastic time and thrombin time were prolonged, fibrinogen concentration was 1 g/l (normal range 1.5–4 g/l) and D-dimer was increased. The blood film showed a number of abnormal white cells, one of which is illustrated in Fig. 5.5.

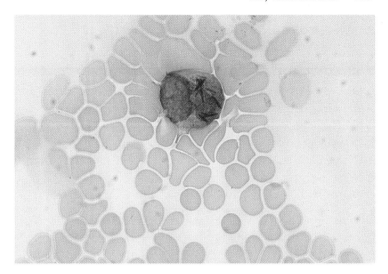

Fig. 5.5 Peripheral blood film (Exercise 5, Q8).

1 What is the abnormal cell?
2 What is the cause of the abnormal coagulation results?
3 What is the most likely diagnosis?
4 What test or tests would you perform to confirm the diagnosis?

Q9 A 60-year-old Englishman presents to his general practitioner with a history of weight loss, dyspnoea on exertion and ankle swelling. He has a good diet. He is found to have an Hb of 8 g/dl, an MCV of 70 fl and an RBC of 3.71 × 10¹²/l.

1 Calculate his PCV, MCH and MCHC.
2 What is the most likely diagnosis?
3 What tests would you do to confirm the diagnosis?
4 What underlying disease would you suspect?

Answers to clinical cases

Q1

1 Leucocytosis with a mixture of mature granulocytes and granulocyte precursors. Few platelets are apparent but the platelet count is high so check more fields.
2 Chronic granulocytic leukaemia (chronic myeloid leukaemia).
3 Cytogenetic analysis for detection of the Philadelphia chromosome [resulting from the translocation t(9;22)(q34;q11)].
4 Neutrophil alkaline phosphatase, serum B_{12} concentration.

Discussion: The clinical history and the height of the WBC indicate that this is some type of leukaemia rather than a reactive condition. Since there are many granulocytes and granulocytic precursors present, this is clearly a myeloid leukaemia, not a lymphoid leukaemia. The large number of mature cells indicate a chronic rather than acute leukaemia. The most likely diagnosis is chronic granulocytic leukaemia (sometimes called chronic myeloid leukaemia). There are no dysplastic features or monocytosis to suggest that this is atypical chronic myeloid leukaemia or chronic myelomonocytic leukaemia.

Cytogenetic analysis to detect the Philadelphia chromosome, resulting from a translocation between chromosomes 9 and 22, would confirm the diagnosis. This test is usually carried out on a bone marrow aspirate. Neutrophil alkaline phosphatase is low in 95% of cases of chronic granulocytic leukaemia and serum B_{12} concentration is elevated but neither of these tests is important if cytogenetic analysis is available.

Q2

1 Anaemia, microcytosis, an NRBC, a sickle cell, a tear-drop poikilocyte, target cells and Pappenheimer bodies.
2 Compound heterozygosity for beta thalassaemia and sickle cell haemoglobin.
3 Haemoglobin electrophoresis and a solubility test for sickle cell haemoglobin. The likely result is that the majority of

haemoglobin will be haemoglobin S with some haemoglobin A₂ and possibly some haemoglobin A or haemoglobin F.

4 Sickle cell trait.

Discussion: Since a sickle cell is present it is clear that the patient has some form of sickle cell disease. Since her mother had beta thalassaemia trait it is not possible for the patient to have sickle cell anaemia (homozygosity for haemoglobin S). The likely diagnosis is compound heterozygosity for beta thalassaemia trait (inherited from her mother) and sickle cell haemoglobin (inherited from her father). The low MCV and the Pappenheimer bodies (the latter consequent on iron overload and hyposplenism) are consistent with this diagnosis. The father must have sickle cell trait (or some other abnormality with at least one β^s gene e.g. sickle cell/haemoglobin C disease). In this particular patient, haemoglobin electrophoresis showed only haemoglobin S as her mother had β^0 thalassaemia trait. If her mother had had β^+ thalassaemia trait then some haemoglobin A would have been present but, in contrast to the findings in sickle cell trait, the percentage of haemoglobin A would have been lower than the percentage of haemoglobin S.

If you gave sickle cell trait as an answer this is wrong. Sickle cell trait does not cause sickle cells in the blood film.

Q3

1 Macrocytosis, irregularly contracted cells and keratocytes.
2 Oxidant-induced haemolytic anaemia caused by dapsone.
3 Heinz body preparation, reticulocyte count and glucose-6-phosphate dehydrogenase (G6PD) assay or red cell folate assay.

Discussion: The blood film changes are typical of oxidant-induced haemolytic anaemia. The keratocytes are caused by the removal of Heinz bodies by the spleen. Dapsone is a known oxidant which commonly causes haemolysis. The macrocytosis is consistent with the reticulocytosis expected in this patient. Her gender and her northern European origin make underlying G6PD deficiency unlikely. The most useful tests would be a Heinz body preparation and a reticulocyte count. The other tests suggested are less likely to be useful since G6PD deficiency is unlikely. If the test is done it is important to relate the result to the reticulocyte count since reticulocytes have a higher concentration of the enzyme than mature erythrocytes. Patients with chronic haemolytic anaemia have an increased need for folic acid and deficiency is therefore possible. However, it is more likely that the macrocytosis is caused by increased numbers of reticulocytes.

Q4

1 Infectious mononucleosis.
2 Primary infection by the Epstein–Barr virus (EBV).
3 A serological test for the heterophile antibody, i.e. a modified Paul–Bunnell test or infectious mononucleosis screening test.

Discussion: This is a typical case of infectious mononucleosis ('glandular fever'). Thrombocytopenia caused by peripheral destruction of platelets is a known complication. Infectious mononucleosis is characterized by the development of a heterophile antibody which agglutinates sheep red cells. The antibody can be identified by a Paul–Bunnell test but this is a labour-intensive test and therefore not usually performed. A rapid screening test which is a modification of the Paul–Bunnell tests (an infectious mononucleosis screening test) is preferred. If the test is negative it should be repeated in 7–10 days. Fig. 3.9 (page 52) shows a typical blood film in this condition.

Q5

1 The blood film shows rouleaux formation and a plasma cell. There is also increased background staining and two red cells appear hypochromic.
2 The most likely diagnosis is multiple myeloma.
3 The two tests most likely to confirm the diagnosis are bone marrow aspiration and serum protein electrophoresis.
4 Renal function may be impaired because of hypercalcaemia, hyperuricaemia and deposition of Bence-Jones protein in the renal tubules.

Discussion: This is a typical case of multiple myeloma. Note that 'myeloma' is not a totally correct answer since solitary myelomas also occur and it is clear that this patient has a disseminated disease.

The two tests suggested are those most likely to confirm the diagnosis. Any paraprotein detected should be quantified. Other tests which may be useful include a radiological survey of the skeleton, examination of the urine for Bence-Jones protein and estimation of the concentration of normal serum immunoglobulins. The erythrocyte sedimentation rate (ESR) is very likely to be elevated in view of the marked rouleaux formation. However, this observation would contribute no diagnostically useful information in this patient and it would be less useful in following the response to treatment than repeated measurements of the concentration of the paraprotein. Note that in this patient the ethnic origin is irrelevant; however, it is always worth noting the ethnic origin because it may suggest a particular diagnosis.

Q6

1 The blood film shows numerous echinocytes (red cell crenation), several fragments and a microspherocyte. Only two platelets are apparent so it is possible that the patient has thrombocytopenia. It is evident that the patient is anaemic and there are some macrocytes.
2 This is a microangiopathic haemolytic anaemia.
3 The most likely diagnosis is haemolytic uraemic syndrome following infection by a verocytotoxin-producing *Escherichia coli*.

Discussion: Thrombotic thrombocytopenic purpura would also be considered in the differential diagnosis of a microangiopathic haemolytic anaemia with a suspicion of thrombocytopenia. However, the history is typical for haemolytic uraemic syndrome and does not mention features suggestive of thrombotic thrombocytopenic purpura such as bruising, purpura or petechiae, fever or neurological abnormalities. The macrocytes are likely to indicate an increased reticulocyte count as a response to the anaemia.

Q7

1 The blood film shows a myeloblast, a hypogranular neutrophil, stomatocytes and tear-drop poikilocytes. The platelet count appears to be reduced but there is a small platelet aggregate at the top of the illustration, so it would be necessary to examine more microscopic fields to confirm the thrombocytopenia.
2 The most likely diagnosis is one of the myelodysplastic syndromes.
3 A bone marrow aspirate is essential for diagnosis.
4 Cytogenetic analysis carried out on the bone marrow aspirate would give information of relevance to prognosis.

Discussion: A bone marrow aspiration is essential for diagnosis. A diagnosis of myelodysplastic syndrome is favoured by the history, which is suggestive of an illness of gradual onset, and, in addition, although there are blast cells in the blood they appear to be infrequent since the total WBC is not elevated. However, without a bone marrow aspirate it is not possible to exclude a diagnosis of acute myeloid leukaemia with associated myelodysplastic features. Cytogenetic analysis gives prognostic information since certain abnormalities (e.g. complex rearrangements and abnormalities of chromosome 7) are associated with a worse prognosis; and if there were any doubt about the prognosis, detection of a clonal cytogenic abnormality could confirm it.

Q8

1 An abnormal promyelocyte containing multiple Auer rods.
2 The tests are indicative of disseminated intravascular coagulation since fibrinogen is reduced and D-dimer (a fibrin degradation product) is increased.
3 Acute hypergranular promyelocytic leukaemia.
4 Bone marrow aspiration and cytogenetic analysis to detect the characteristic translocation, t(15;17)(q22;q21).

Discussion: The combination of disseminated intravascular coagulation and an abnormal promyelocyte with multiple Auer rods suggests a diagnosis of acute myeloid leukaemia of the hypergranular promyelocytic type (M3 acute myeloid leukaemia). It is not uncommon for this type of leukaemia to present with a marked reduction of the platelet count but without severe anaemia or leucocytosis. Disseminated intravascular coagulation is characteristic of this subtype of acute myeloid leukaemia. Detection of the t(15;17) translocation confirms the diagnosis. If it is not detected, molecular analysis for detection of the *PML-RARA* fusion gene is indicated. Because of the frequency of disseminated intravascular coagulation, it is important to be alert to the possibility of this diagnosis and to confirm it as a matter of urgency so that specific treatment can be started.

Q9

1 The PCV is 0.26, the MCH 21.5 pg and the MCHC 31.0 g/dl. If you cannot remember the relevant formulae, they can be found on page 20.
2 Iron deficiency.
3 The diagnosis could be confirmed either by demonstrating a low serum ferritin concentration or by demonstrating both a reduced serum iron concentration and either an elevated total iron binding capacity or an elevated transferrin concentration.
4 Occult gastrointestinal haemorrhage, e.g. due to carcinoma of the colon or diverticular disease.

Discussion: The indices are typical of iron deficiency and the history, although non-specific, is consistent with this. In a middle-aged Englishman whose diet is normal this is most probably due to occult gastrointestinal haemorrhage, either from the large bowel or from the stomach. Biochemical tests on the blood are likely to confirm the diagnosis of iron deficiency and it is unlikely that a bone marrow aspiration would be needed for confirmation in this patient. It is very important to identify the underlying cause, since iron deficiency anaemia can be the presenting feature of an otherwise occult gastrointestinal malignancy.

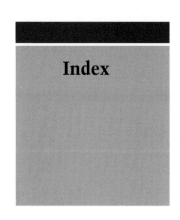

Index